THE POWER CYCLE

TIME EFFICIENT CYCLED TRAINING FOR STRENGTH, MUSCLE SIZE, AND FITNESS.

By
Collier Todd Hageman

This book is dedicated to the best trainer and teacher in the business, Phil Evanisko. On behalf of myself and the countless people you've helped over the years, thank you for everything my friend.

A special note of gratitude to the staff and members of my gym in Falls Church, Virginia. I can't imagine a better place to work or train, or a better bunch of people to do it with. Also to my clients and friends at Vinson Hall in McLean, Virginia. You motivate and inspire me and make it possible for me to make a living doing something I enjoy immensely. From my heart I thank you.

PREFACE

The methodology and general theory
described herein is useful to anyone interested
in increasing their strength levels and general health and fitness,
but it is essential it be implemented using good and
well-maintained equipment. Safety first!

CYCLED TRAINING

WHY WEIGHT TRAIN? HOW DO YOU BUILD MUSCLE?

Weight training is one of the most popular forms of exercise because it is the single most effective and efficient way to get bigger and stronger, provided it is done properly. Having a powerful and muscular physique not only looks great, it *feels* great, and not just physically but mentally and emotionally as well. It is a boost to self confidence, vitality, and health in general.

Increasing your functional strength and muscle mass only becomes more important with age, not less. We need to try to build our muscles as Father Time tries to rob us of them, but the same workout that built and maintained our strength when we are in our twenties won't be suitable for this purpose when we are in our fifties, sixties, and beyond. When you lose muscle *everything* becomes more difficult. If you build plenty of muscle before middle age, you'll have some money in the bank, so to speak, when age starts trying to whittle away at it. This is not to say that you can't build muscle and strength once youth fades. I give some true accounts in this book that prove the opposite. It is always possible to improve, but you have to train smarter as you get older, and cycled training is a valuable tool for this. It is self-paced, adaptable, dynamic, and effective.

There is also an indirect but very real fat-loss/weight-control benefit to weight training, besides just the calories consumed working out. Every pound of muscle you have on your frame metabolizes about fifty calories a day, even if you do nothing but lie in bed all day. Of course when you're active this figure becomes much higher. Muscle raises your metabolic rate and makes your body a more efficient calorie processor, and because of this muscular people also have an advantage in staying lean. This seems monumentally unfair, but that's the way it is.

To train with efficiency and purpose requires a plan. Unfortunately most people begin weight training with no clear plan in mind, and this can cause them to waste lots of precious time and effort. Any exercise, provided it is done safely, is better than none at all, and so these folks will initially enjoy some benefit. Some eventually learn what works and they develop or adopt a good training plan, but many others continue to weight train regularly but fruitlessly, day in, day out, month after month, gaining little or no muscle mass and precious little strength.

You know who I mean. You've seen them. In fact you might *be* them – the guy or gal who shows up at the gym religiously and grits it out through a workout that lasts an hour and a half, or two, or even longer. Often they bang their way through the same routine, in the same order, with the same weight, for the same number of reps and sets, usually topping it with an interminably long cardio session, day in, day out, sometimes for years on end, yet never improve. If you ask why they don't vary their routine or challenge themselves with something different, their answer will be something along the lines of "because this is the way I've always done it!"

And of course this is exactly the reason why they never improve. Another factor may be that they are exercise addicts and train too much. Train too much? Some of you understand this concept, but to some it will sound like heresy. Make a note – we'll look at this later. If you know someone like this, do them a favor and tell them about this method. Don't be surprised if your words fall on deaf ears however. Its likely that their dead-end workout is hopelessly ingrained upon their psyche, but at least you have presented them with an option, perhaps made them think.

Many people, primarily female, approach me saying they don't want to build muscle, they 'just want to do toning'. Make no mistake; toning **is** muscle building. It is impossible to make a muscle harder and more shapely without building it. Without chemical help women generally cannot put on muscle mass to the extent that is possible for men, as they do not have the level of testosterone that men do, but women do have some testosterone, just as men have some estrogen. I have trained women who developed high levels of strength, using training cycles similar to those I use with men, with appropriate adjustments according to their own abilities and goals.

Needless to say, in achieving strength they also achieved excellent 'muscle tone', though their training goes beyond that. Although they have to train smarter and more diligently for their strength and muscle than most men, they are by and large quite feminine, some even beautiful. One of the best things about cycled training is that it is endlessly adaptable and can be adjusted simply and readily to each individual, regardless of sex, age, body type, and physical condition.

I trained one of my most memorable clients, Liliane DeRouas, with the cycled training method. She is an active and athletic woman who swims, bicycles and plays tennis, but when I met her she did no weight training. In a year and a half of diligent training with this method her strength increased to a point that she was capable of strict leg presses, with a full range of motion on a plate-loaded forty-five degree leg press machine, with four hundred eighty-five pounds for sets of twelve reps, and she was ready for an increase when she moved from the area. Guys would stop and watch, some with amazement, some with embarrassment, when she did this. She more than tripled the functional strength of her legs with cycled training. She more than doubled her upper body strength.

She weighs about one hundred forty-five pounds. She was fifty-seven years old when I trained her. She is every inch a lady and turned heads when she entered the gym. Her greatest asset, other than glowing good health and marvelous sense of humor, is her amazing attitude. She is always willing to push herself to excel and never told me that she couldn't do something. "Let me try!" is her mantra. Incidentally, Liliane has arthritis. One of the most effective treatments for this potentially debilitating condition is, yes, weight training.

There are two points to this. First, ladies don't be afraid of having muscles! A strong and muscular physique, within reason, looks good on anyone. Second, our greatest limitations are those we place on ourselves. Most of them exist only in our minds. Arnold Schwarzenegger has stated this repeatedly throughout his life and he hasn't done too badly for himself, especially considering his modest beginnings.

I have trained a number of people who were at first mortified at the prospect of gaining a scant half pound, even if it were solid muscle. Though it is more often true of women there are plenty of men who are fixated, obsessive even, about their weight, and can't pass a scale without jumping on to check it, even several times a day. Please divest yourself of the notion that there is ONE weight you should be. You have a *weight range,* and the larger framed a person is the larger this range may be. It isn't unusual for a man over two hundred pounds to fluctuate in weight across a range of four to ten pounds, even in a single day, depending on food and water intake, physical activities, and - excuse me - how 'regular' they are. I don't refer to the unfortunates who suffer from thyroid troubles, or some other clinical malady that causes them to be overweight, though exercise is even more important for them. My typical *weight range* is from two hundred fifteen pounds to two hundred twenty-four pounds, though it does dip below this occasionally in the summer when I'm outdoors more, pursuing other fitness activities besides weight training.

Some doctors continue to do people great disservice by adhering strictly to the height/weight table. I've had the experience, more than once, of weighing in during a visit to a doctor and being then told that I was overweight, once I was even called obese, because I am five feet ten inches tall and weigh in the neighborhood of two hundred twenty pounds. They paid NO attention whatever to the fact that my bodyfat has been at or below - sometimes way below - twelve percent for over twenty years, and that I have a thirty-three inch waist. One internist (the one that pronounced me obese) informed me that I was supposed to weigh "no more than one hundred sixty-eight pounds." He did not examine me before saying this. In fact he barely looked at me. He referred only to a graph on a clipboard. For the record, I haven't weighed a hundred and sixty-eight pounds since I was twelve years old, and have never been fat. I've heard many stories just like this from people who weight train regularly.

If you are a numbers-oriented person and need figures to go by then use your bodyfat and circumferential measurements. These, taken every three months, will give a weight trainer a more realistic and accurate assessment of overall fitness than numbers on a bathroom scale. It IS a good idea to weigh yourself ONCE a week. Pick a day and hour and do it at the same time every week, say, noon every Saturday, in the same apparel, or without apparel. Following this is also a much more realistic and practical way of tracking your weight and assessing changes in your body as you continue to improve as a result of your workouts. Just don't be put off when it climbs as you gain muscle.

However, if you are still afraid of gaining muscle in spite of my exhortations, and just want to go through the motions of weight training without really challenging yourself, and say you are 'toning', then please don't waste any more time on this book. Instead, I recommend you take up running and do calisthenics at home, then take the money you save by not purchasing a gym membership or home equipment and invest it in a good set of orthotics. You may need them.

The method outlined in this manual, cycled training, is simple and it works. Please note, I said simple, NOT easy. Banish that word from your lexicon because an easy workout is not a workout. Building strength and muscle mass is a lot of hard work, but it is *productive* hard work and cycled training makes it more productive and efficient.

I do not take the position that cycled training is the only valid training method. Far from it. There are several, and I encourage you to try any and all that interest you. Your experience will be much the same as mine in that you'll find that some work for you and some don't. Other people will get results from things that you didn't profit from at all, and vice versa. Personally, I love learning about and trying new techniques, but I have always come back to cycled training. It is still the basis for all my workouts.

I have put on an average of three pounds of solid muscle a year with this method, and I am what is referred to as a hard gainer. To many this may seem a paltry amount, but if you multiply that by the twenty-five years I have weight-trained you'll see that it is not at all insignificant.

If you've never weight-trained, or are coming off a significant layoff, its likely you'll gain more than this the first year. Most people's initial strength increases and muscular weight gains are the greatest they ever experience. For example, if you are a man not yet in middle age, average sized, with a medium frame, and apply yourself diligently to this method, you can expect a gain of eight to twelve pounds your first year. Women will experience less, perhaps half this, due primarily to the testosterone factor discussed earlier.

Very occasionally I've seen people gain more than eight to twelve pounds naturally (i.e. without pharmaceutical help) in their first year of regular training, but they were exceptional. They were very driven and worked out with greater intensity than most folks can muster, and/or they were just naturally *mesomorphic* and gained muscle mass quicker and easier than most people. I envy these individuals but, alas, am not one of them. I've labored long and hard for every ounce of muscle I've put on my frame, but cycled training has kept my gains coming steadily for several years, though naturally with a temporary plateau once in a great while.

Initially however you will experience a period where you will have strength gains, sometimes quite dramatic ones, long before you start to notice visible changes in your physique. This is due to something called enervation, or an increase in, as I call it, nerve strength. This concept is important and deserves further attention:

A large part of physical power lies not in the muscles but in the nerves. You probably have seen someone who was strong all out of proportion with their size. They may not even be particularly muscular, but they can move some serious weight. They have superior enervation.

The number of nerves stimulating any muscle is genetically determined and won't be increased by any amount of weight training. Some people have more than others. As far as physical strength and power go they are lucky indeed.

When you first begin a certain lift, only the minimum number of muscle fibers necessary will be stimulated by the nerves to contract to move that amount of weight. As you continue to perform that movement in your workouts over a period of time, adding more weight, more muscle fibers are stimulated by more nerves to perform the more demanding workload. This is referred to as recruitment. It also occurs during a single set as muscle fibers become fatigued. Your body becomes better at this recruitment with repetition and practice and this is the reason, especially in the beginning phase of a weight training program, that you may occasionally experience the odd phenomena of a second or even third set being easier than the first.

For this reason I have always found it advantageous before any lift to do a set of twelve to fifteen repetitions with an empty bar or unloaded apparatus, or even just move my limbs through the range of motion required by that movement. This will help the enervation of your muscles for that lift, and give a little warmup to them and the involved joints as well.

I have heard it said that the 'signal strength' and efficiency of the electrical impulses traveling along the nerves can be improved by weight training as well. I believe that this could well be possible though I don't personally know of any clinical studies that prove it. Also, simply becoming familiar with the way a certain movement feels, and training your nerves and muscles to perform it properly, will naturally result in an ability to perform it with more weight. This is all a part of nerve strength, and initially this increases much more quickly than the rate at which muscle fibers grow larger.

And when your muscles grow, it is the existing muscle

fibers getting larger. This is called *hypertrophy*. The number of fibers does not increase. That is called *hyperplasia* and has not been proven to be a natural occurrence in humans. I say natural occurrence because there is some evidence that it can occur with the help of regular injections of Human Growth Hormone (HGH) combined with heavy workouts. It does happen naturally in certain animals under certain conditions. For example racehorses commonly exhibit it.

When your muscles do start to actually grow larger, others will notice it before you do. For this reason it is useful to have photos taken of yourself, in brief workout attire, when you begin a weight training program, and again every four to six months in the same attire. Photos don't lie, and this way you will have incontrovertible evidence of your improvement.

Make no mistake, when you have been training for a few years a gain of three pounds of solid muscle in a single year is a good amount, contrary to some supplement ads claiming that gains of ten, twenty, or even more pounds of solid muscle are possible, even easy, in ridiculously short periods of time, with use of their product. Please believe me, the only substances capable of producing anything even remotely like these rapid and dramatic gains are not legal without a prescription.

CREATINE

A substance that in certain circumstances can enable some relatively rapid gains is creatine. I'll elaborate on this here, as creatine can be a useful supplement and is wildly popular. For those seeking muscle size and strength creatine has three desirable effects.

1) It enables your muscles to contract with more force. This is due to its positive effect on your body's energy production and the ATP cycle within the mitochondria of your cells. Quite literally it makes you stronger. While you're on it.

2) It increases protein synthesis within the muscles. It enables

you to build muscle tissue more easily. A little.

3) It causes greater water retention in the cells. As opposed to other types of water retention this is not a bad thing. An increase in *intercellular* water in the muscles means larger muscles. However this effect is temporary.

Red meat, particularly beef, is the best dietary source of creatine. Thus, vegetarians or those who don't eat red meat, and don't have as much creatine in their bodies to begin with, can experience some good weight and strength gains when first taking it, and an occasional cycle of creatine will be of some benefit to most people who weight train, vegetarian or not.

It should be done only in cycles. That is, do it for several weeks then go off of it for a similar length of time. The first time I did a cycle of creatine my strength increased noticeably and I am no vegetarian. But I was quite enthused about trying it so I believe that much of the boost I received was psychological, and I've never had gains from it as spectacular as those. But the fact remains that, for whatever reason, all my lifts increased. I like getting stronger and if a psychological factor was responsible for a large part of this dramatic strength increase, well, that is okay with me.

In a few of my lifts the increase was only ten pounds, but in several it was much more. My workout weight on a ten degree flye machine went from one hundred eighty pounds to two hundred fifty pounds, and I could have done more but this was the maximum possible on that particular machine.

While some people (again, usually vegetarians) also experience a dramatic increase in muscle size and a solid weight gain along with this strengthening effect, I did not. My gain in bodyweight was about five pounds, much of which eventually disappeared when I stopped taking creatine. This was probably due to the water retention effect, but because it does increase the assimilation of protein into muscles, some part of a size/weight gain should be lasting. In my experience it was only a small part, although because it allowed me to train harder with heavier weights it did contribute to a lasting strength gain. My experience with creatine is not atypical. I don't believe that most people trying it will ever experience more than a ten pound weight gain due to creatine, no matter what brand or formulation, and probably not even this much.

Three considerations about creatine, should you choose to try it. The first is to drink plenty of water. Inadequate water intake causes a metabolite of creatine called creatinine to build up in your system, causing muscle weakness. Eventually there will be other negative effects. Secondly, some people find that creatine causes them intestinal distress and/or bloating. This may be mild and disappear once you get used to taking it, or it can be more severe and lasting and preclude using it altogether. Some people simply cannot take creatine. Thirdly, get the best creatine you can find. There is huge difference in quality and purity between different brands. With some of it you'd be better off eating dirt. There are also some formulations that contain creatine that is good enough, but then combine it with other substances that are completely unneeded. One popular formulation that comes to mind gives you more than twenty grams of *sugar* per serving.

Do your research and look for an independent laboratory analysis proving one hundred percent pure creatine monohydrate. There are certain brands that always meet this benchmark. I won't advertise any particular brand of creatine or other supplements in this manual but suffice to say you should stick with familiar brands known for quality. Good creatine is not cheap, but you get what you pay for with this stuff. *Caveat emptor.*

BODY TYPES

Some may be unfamiliar with the term *mesomorphic* I used earlier. Allow me to here define and clarify this. There are three basic body types: mesomorphic, endomorphic, and ectomorphic.

A *mesomorph* is a person naturally gifted with a

predominantly muscular physique, generally with broad shoulders, narrow hips and waist. They can build muscle relatively easily. Typically they have medium to low bodyfat levels and are inclined to be active, strong, and energetic. They most obvious example of this bodytype is what comes to mind when we think of a professional bodybuilder.

An *endomorph* is a person that we would commonly refer to as 'big-boned' or less kindly, 'dumpy'. These folks gain weight easily, tending toward obesity, and generally have thick torsos, wide hips, and a large waistline. Often they actually possess very large muscles but they probably won't be visible because of bodyfat levels in the high to very high range. They can also possess significant strength and power, but typically have low energy levels. A good albeit extreme example of this bodytype is a sumo wrestler. I think there can be little argument that mighty Paul Anderson, the strongest man in recent history, at five feet nine inches tall and at one time weighing in the neighborhood of three hundred eighty pounds was endomorphic, though he obviously had an enormous mesomorphic component also. Atypically Paul did *not* have low energy levels. In fact he was a very energetic man and capable of surprising athleticism. More on these combination bodytypes in a moment.

An *ectomorph* has naturally low bodyfat and typically is what we would call 'small-boned'. They are skinny, simply put, and are not naturally powerful. Typically they have a lot of nervous energy and may be prone to hyperactivity. Some ectomorphs are actually very athletic. For example many, probably most, marathoners are ectomorphic. I have trained ectomorphs that built good, quality muscle and became quite strong for their size, but this only came at the expense of lots of sweat and time.

All this being said, most people are not pure examples of any one of these three basic bodytypes, but combinations of two, or possibly even all three of them. For example surely the strongest, most powerful bodytype is neither a purely mesomorphic or endomorphic type, but a combination of these called a meso-endomorph. Think of the new breed of NFL linemen with gigantic frames, huge limbs, big joints and bones, but without a huge gut, and only medium to high medium bodyfat. Many of them are near or over the three hundred pound mark but aren't obese, and some of them can **run**.

Many smaller-framed bodybuilders are ecto-mesomorphs and exhibit excellent muscle definition due to their low bodyfat. There are rare ecto-mesomorphs that possess strength that would be impossible to a purely ectomorphic type. My old training partner Dean Tait is definitely one of these and consistently outlifts much larger men, myself included - at least, on some lifts. Ray Koury is another good example of a very strong ecto-mesomorph. At six feet one, and one hundred seventy-five pounds, Ray is capable of a five hundred pound squat for reps.

Ray is a man devoted to a fitness lifestyle. In addition to weight training religiously he plays semi-pro basketball, runs daily, is a martial artist, a doctor of chiropractic and a vegetarian. An interesting, supremely healthy, and well-rounded man.

A few years ago somatotyping was all the rage. This was a method of classifying a physique by assigning a numerical ranking, from one to seven, (before you ask – I do not know why a seven point scale rather than a ten point scale is used) according to how strongly a person's physique exhibits characteristics of each of the three basic types. For example, someone exhibiting only some of the burliness of an endomorph, with all the muscularity and narrow waist of a mesomorph, and with only the naturally low bodyfat of an ectomorph might be given a ranking of 2-7-2 as his somatotype. An interesting tool, perhaps useful for trainers or bodybuilding judges. Incidentally, someone with this particular somatotype ranking would have great natural gifts to succeed as a bodybuilder or strength athlete.

While it is impossible to change your genes, it is possible to change your somatotype ranking and, to an extent, even your bodytype. I know of individuals who were assuredly endomorphs, but through lots of weight training and attention to their nutrition could now rightly only be referred to as mesomorphic, though it is arguable that they are in fact now an endo-mesomorph.

My friend Trenton Brown is a wonderful example of this. In a year and a half he turned his slack three hundred forty pound body into a muscular and lean two hundred thirty pound training *machine*. Don't **even** get between him and the heavy bag when he slips on his sparring gloves.

Theoretically, an endomorph or a mesomorph could be turned into an ectomorph through starvation dieting or some other terrible wasting condition, God forbid.

Through lots of heavy workouts using cycled training I changed my nearly ectomorphic body from a skinny one hundred fifty pounds to a mesomorphic, rock-solid two hundred twenty pounds and kept my bodyfat at or below twelve percent - low for a man my age. This is a seventy pound gain of mostly muscle, but it hardly occurred overnight. The gains that come with cycled training are very real and come steadily and regularly but, as with any routine, you will eventually plateau. There are several techniques that work quite well for jump-starting your progress when this happens, and they can be temporarily assimilated into your training cycle quite easily. These are addressed in a later section.

I'm not a doctor, though you'd think so to listen to the litany of medical and physical conditions that people seek out my advice on. I generally just listen and this is usually enough. But I am merely a strength trainer. I love lifting weights more than any other type of exercise. That is what I do the most of, know the most about, and what I can assist others with best.

CARDIO

For this reason, if cardio is the most important type of training to you (and that's fine if it is), you should consult a good running coach, marathoner, or aerobics instructor. That is not my field of expertise and this book is not for that purpose.

On the other hand, I would never minimize the importance of this form of exercise, and so will write of its more salient points as it pertains to general fitness and how it can impact strength training, both positively and negatively.

Powerful muscles will improve your endurance, and benefit your cardio training and performance. They enable your body to use oxygen and pump blood more efficiently. Conversely, there is absolutely no doubt that a strong healthy heart, strong lungs, and good stamina will benefit your weight training.

A good book on this subject is <u>Peripheral Heart Action,</u> by George Miller. I know George and he is in phenomenal shape, not even considering the fact that he is over seventy years old. He is just a man in great shape, period, and his clear and well-written book is well worth reading.

For those whose priority is gaining strength and muscle mass, three cardio sessions thirty to forty-five minutes long per week, wherein your heart rate hits sixty-five to eighty-five percent of your maximum, will suffice. The layman's rule of thumb for calculating your maximum heart rate is to start with the base figure two hundred ten, subtract fifty percent of your age, subtract five percent of your weight, plus four if you're a male, plus zero if you're female.

You can benefit from this level of cardio training and generally not impact your weight training negatively. Its wonderful to have great stamina or to have great power, but its better to possess both, and both types of training are necessary to achieve and maintain balanced fitness.

However, if you're unable to gain strength and muscle mass, it may be that your level of cardio/aerobic training is too great. If this is you, please at least consider decreasing the frequency and duration of your cardio sessions.

Some do this type of training purely for the health benefits to their circulatory and respiratory systems. Controlling their weight simply is not their need or priority, but many who engage regularly in cardio/aerobic exercise do so with their primary goal being to lower or maintain their bodyfat level. If this is you then incorporate cardio into your cycled training regimen in the fashion described below.

On days when you do both a weight training and a cardio training workout it is better to weight train first *then* do your cardio, exactly the opposite of how most people do it. I believe most folks simply think it is easier to do cardio first because they rely on it as a warmup for their weight training. This is *less* efficient, not more, from both a time and a fat loss standpoint.

There is something called the aerobic threshold. This refers to the point at which your body has exhausted its ready fuel stores – muscle glycogen – and begins to metabolize bodyfat for fuel. In adults this happens after about twenty minutes of sustained aerobic exercise, on an empty stomach. If you eat and then do your cardio workout, your body will be manufacturing muscle glycogen while it is using it, and you may never reach that aerobic threshold in that workout. You will still be using up calories of course, but not calories from stored bodyfat.

Weight training does not use muscle glycogen at the rate that vigorous aerobic activity does, but it does use some. It must. Every single contraction of every muscle uses glycogen to power it, from running to doing heavy squats to blinking your eyelids. So, if you perform a half hour of cycled training (all you need in one workout with this training method), then begin your cardio immediately afterwards, you'll hit that aerobic threshold much sooner than the twenty minute mark. It is impossible to say how much sooner, so many are the variables affecting this from individual to individual and from workout to workout, but it **will** be sooner. You could then do a half hour of cardio and be done with your total workout in an hour, and you will have metabolized more fat (not total calories) than if you had merely done it in the reverse order for the same amounts of time.

This being said, do not skip a warmup because it involves cardio/aerobic exercise. Yes, it will add to the time you must spend in the gym, but its when people skip warming up that they start experiencing muscle pulls, injuries to connective tissues, even tears. Be safe and always, **always** warm up and stretch beforehand.

It is also more efficient, again purely from a fat-loss standpoint, to do this workout as early in the day as possible. Cardio/aerobic exercise raises your metabolic rate and it does not plummet as soon as you stop, but continues to be higher for quite some time afterward, eventually returning to normal. So, all else being equal, you have metabolized more calories by the time you fall asleep (when your metabolic rate really plummets) the day you do this workout at seven AM versus the day you do it at seven PM.

You often hear the buzz in spas and aerobics studios, even gyms: "You can't do too much cardio!" Consider the source. This is usually uttered by scrawny people who can run like a deer but couldn't curl a thirty pound dumbbell to save their lives. Believe me, if your focus is gaining strength and muscle mass, it is VERY possible to do too much cardio. Too much cardio/aerobic exercise will take energy, calories, and time that should go to your weight training. It can cause you to plateau. Even worse than this, it can cause your body to cannibalize your hard-earned muscle tissue for fuel. Thats right, too much cardio can lead to muscle *shrinkage* and weakness. Exercise addicts are much more commonly seen on the treadmill than in the squat rack, though it does occur. A true and extreme example of 'too much cardio' follows.

A lady once approached me wanting me to train her in a fashion to increase her muscle mass because her doctor had ordered her to gain weight. She was very distressed at the prospect of gaining any weight at all but said she would try since it was doctor's orders. However she insisted that it be "only solid muscle, absolutely no fat," This is extremely difficult to do. In fact, its virtually impossible.

She was an intelligent and accomplished woman, an attorney, in her late forties, five and a half feet tall and weighed *seventy-five pounds*. During the fitness evaluation I always do before training any client, I found that she could not curl a pair of three pound dumbbells for a full set of ten reps, yet she was adamant about starting a *powerlifting* program. For those unfamiliar with powerlifting, it requires extremely demanding training with maximum weights, and on a cycle of sorts interestingly enough. She'd read that powerlifting is a good way to gain muscle, and insisted that she could handle it because she was "obviously in great shape" because she ran twelve miles every day and had "a healthy diet".

Upon further query I found that her "healthy diet" was in total, two cans of a liquid meal replacement formula and a small salad every day, plus lots of water. I desired to the depths of my heart to help her, but her problems went beyond what strength training could address. Weight training, as she insisted on doing it, would've done irreparable harm to her already damaged body.

Strangely, she was very forthcoming about a host of ailments she suffered due to the stresses that running put on her frail and eroded skeleton. Yet in the next breath she steadfastly maintained that she was "in great shape" and absolutely refused to entertain the idea of stopping or even cutting down on the running that essentially was killing her. In fact when I told her this was prerequisite to me training her she became very troubled and agitated by the notion. In the end, not only could I do nothing for her, I strongly felt that medical/psychiatric help was required and I told her this as tactfully and considerately as possible.

She agreed with me, at least to my face, but I never saw her in the gym again. I could do nothing else but say a silent prayer for her. Without a doubt, an example of "too much cardio".

I wish I had a dollar for every time someone has told me "I walk/run, so I don't need weight training for my legs. I just need to do upper body stuff." Or "Oh, I do the elliptical cross-trainer so I don't need to weight train." **Arrgh!** Let me be clear on this point. Cardio/aerobic exercise, be it walking, running, rowing, using an elliptical cross-trainer, bicycling, swimming, high-kicking with the Rockettes for two solid hours a day, whatever, is NOT a substitute for weight training! Cardio builds endurance and stamina, certainly important parts of fitness, but it is of very little benefit in building actual muscle power, and no use at whatever in adding muscle *size.*

A rare exception to this, and I draw upon my first-hand experience with geriatrics, is in a case where an individual does NOTHING for exercise, and has not for a long while. In this sorry state, it is possible for a person to experience some muscle strengthening and perhaps even regain a tiny bit of muscle mass from walking or pedaling an exercise bike. This improvement is slight and does not continue for long. Essentially what they are doing is counteracting muscle atrophy. This sad but thankfully uncommon situation aside, walking, running, whatever, will NOT increase the power or size of any of your skeletal muscles. As stated before, it will result in actual muscle shrinkage if done to excess, as in the tragic and profound example of the lady above, when the body consumes its own tissues to sustain itself.

Runners and other endurance athletes commonly experience this, though thankfully to a more limited degree. When their glycogen stores are exhausted, and because they generally have such low bodyfat, their body starts to metabolize muscle protein for fuel. Think of your typical marathoner. What do their legs look like? Do they have large, shapely muscles? No, they have legs with thin, knotty, stringy muscles. They're rock-hard, but they are *small*, mostly because of this self-cannibalization effect. They are capable however, of moving up and down like pistons while bearing the subject's body weight, albeit within a very limited range of motion, for twenty six point two miles, an accomplishment that I will not denigrate.

Now think of a bodybuilder that is capable of a four, or even five hundred pound squat for reps. Big muscles as hard as iron, and beautifully shaped as well. But can they run a marathon? A ten k? Are they capable of being competitive in endurance sports? Probably not, although I do know of a few exceptions to this.

An acquaintance of mine, Rick Bucinell, can squat four

hundred five pounds for three sets of *twenty* reps, remarkable in terms of both power and stamina. He has set amateur world records in both the snatch and the clean and jerk. He also engages in long distance bicycle riding. Arnold Schwarzenegger and Tom Platz, both of whom possessed huge, hyper-developed legs, have said they enjoy distance running. There are these rare individuals capable of both. Funny, but these exceptions are weight lifters that also sometimes engage in endurance sports, not marathoners who also occasionally lift weights. Hmmm.

For the record, let me state that anyone that finishes a marathon is a winner in my book and certainly has my respect. They are incredible athletes. Period.

These are illustrations of the difference between strength and power. Certainly the two are closely related, but strength is a broad term encompassing muscle stamina, cardiovascular endurance, and the ability to apply force with your muscles. Power is the ability to move a given weight over a given range in a given time, a crucial part of strength, but only a part. Cycled training has a positive effect on both.

The beauty of the cycled method is that it can be adapted to be useful for beginning, intermediate, or advanced weight trainers. Marathoners benefit from it, as do housewives, as do football players. It also works for all age groups, requiring only adapting the amount of weight used in any lift to fit any of these different levels and abilities, but this, like the entire program, is simplicity itself. One simple concept, the three sets of ten rule, discussed in the chapter entitled 'Training Cycles', covers this for everyone.

AGE & STRENGTH TRAINING

While I certainly advocate weight training for adolescents, especially in these times when obesity and other ailments caused by inactivity (the 'politically correct' term for *laziness*) are epidemic in kids, under **no** circumstances do I advocate any training involving maximum lifts for those younger than sixteen, and preferably eighteen. The still-pliable bones of those younger than this could be injured by the stresses involved in heavy training. Great improvements in both strength and muscle size can be realized by those younger than this with the cycled method, starting at a minimum age of thirteen.

I say this with utter sincerity while fully cognizant of the utter futility of recommending that teenage boys not test their strength. Its like telling people not to have sex. They'll do it anyway. Its really only natural that anyone involved with weight training, particularly young boys, will want to test themselves, explore the limits of their strength, and show off a bit, frankly. This should only be done under the guidance and close supervision of a strength coach, trainer, phys-ed teacher or simply an experienced and willing adult lifter that knows proper form. And I do mean that <u>knows</u> <u>proper</u> form.

I strongly advocate the use of weight machines for this type of adolescent training and testing. While free weights are generally superior to machines in producing overall size and strength gains, machines are better for isolating certain muscles and muscle groups and are inherently safer than free weights. **Safety is *always* the most important thing in any training**.

On the other end of the age spectrum, I have personally witnessed the doubling, tripling, and in one case, the quadrupling of functional strength in senior citizens. To increase your functional strength four hundred percent is an enormous accomplishment. If I could do this now I could be a superhero.

The other important, no, *crucial,* but often ignored type of exercise is <u>stretching</u>. If you can't move smoothly, with agility, over a full range of motion, and without pain, what good is all the strength and stamina in the world? This also becomes increasingly important as we age, and I will even go so far as to say perhaps even more so than either aerobic or anaerobic exercise. I have seen scores of seniors who appeared healthy but actually suffered various degrees of disability, some quite severe, simply because they had been inactive, and grown stiff from not moving their joints and muscles through a full range of motion regularly. I am not speaking of cases of people suffering from degenerative disease beyond their control. I am speaking of people who have *crippled themselves* through inactivity and not stretching.

I hold a stretching class twice a week and am always amazed by the flexibility and suppleness exhibited by my friend Helen Anderson. She is a lovely lady well into her eighties, who looks sixty, and who can achieve positions and has a range of motion that exceeds my own ability, and I'm considered quite limber. She credits many years of yoga for this. I've seen many other yoga practitioners demonstrate remarkable flexibility and good overall health and I'm convinced of its efficacy. Based on this, if you have the time and inclination, I heartily recommend yoga.

Another practice that I am positive is beneficial, not only to achieving and maintaining flexibility, but to general fitness and strength, is Tai Chi. I am by no means a Tai Chi expert, though I do assist and lead seniors in an elementary Tai Chi class once a week. When first undertaking this I was shocked at the effort that an hour of this slow, gentle method requires and the effect it had. I cannot definitely say that there was a direct cause and effect relationship, but the fact is that after taking up Tai Chi I enjoyed a period wherein my strength increased noticeably.

A personal note here. Working with geriatrics is one of the most rewarding things I've ever done and I recommend it whole-heartedly, in any way that you can be of service. Old folks are a treasure and are the ones who have made our lives possible. They are our roots, bridges to our past, and the village elders of our time. Bringing a little joy into their sometimes lonely lives and being of help to them is something you should experience. I honestly feel its my duty, but its never a burden. In fact, it is a privilege. My secret is that, while I absolutely do help them and love doing it, I benefit more from their wisdom, humor, experience, and sage counsel than they do from me sharing my knowledge.

One of the main symptoms of aging is loss of muscle

mass and functional strength. The tragedy here is that it is, to a great extent, avoidable. The way to avoid it is through exercise and weight training. Let me relate the best example of this that I personally know of.

I am proud to be friends with Mr. Hezekiah Daniel. This old Georgia gentleman grew strong as a young man working as a blacksmith and clearing timber for farmland with an axe and a team of horses. You won't meet many these days who have done harder physical work than this. Though country strong from an early age, he didn't even start regular weight training until the age of sixty-four at the encouragement of his son, an accomplished bodybuilder.

Shortly after I met him he participated in an amateur bodybuilding contest. Need I say he was the oldest man to enter? This contest had no grand masters or ultra masters divisions because he was put in the masters division, for those age forty and above. This put him in direct competition with several men more than *thirty years younger* than he was. He won. Decisively. And, proving it was no fluke, he went on to repeat this in another amateur contest a few months later. Hezekiah is a modest and quiet man, but when I got to know him better I learned that he already had over a dozen first place trophies at that time.

As he continued to win them, we proudly displayed his trophies at the gym. I was flattered yet humbled when members asked if the trophies were mine. I sheepishly had to tell them thanks but no, they belonged to the seventy-two year old man over at the squat rack.

Bodybuilders benefit greatly from the cycled training method, and while power lifters adhere to their own particular training regimen, culminating in a max lift only in competition, they can also benefit from periodic implementation of this method. Olympic style lifters find it a natural. For most, those simply interested in getting bigger, stronger, and more fit, it is especially valuable and this is who will initially experience the greatest benefit.

The methodology of this type of training has three basic

aspects. They are: training frequency, training divisions, and training cycles. In very basic terms this means how many sets and reps you do, the actual lifts you must do, and how often you lift. Please read this manual to the end before implementing any of the techniques and/or lifts outlined. It is important that you fully understand what these all entail before embarking on a cycled training regimen.

BEFORE YOU START

There are some requirements for this regimen. Foremostly, if you have any medical condition or debility, or have been inactive for a long while, a doctors examination or consultation is essential. If you are cleared for vigorous training you next need a comprehensive array of home equipment, or a gym membership.

Let me be clear: A barbell and a bench, while excellent and essential strength training tools, are not adequate for a thorough cycled training workout. On the other hand, you don't *need* a membership at a high dollar 'spa' or 'health club' either. Shop around in your area. Look in the phone book under 'gym'. In some areas the YMCA is the best deal in town, in others it is not. There is nothing really wrong with a fancy workout facility, but don't let neon lights and pretty chrome dumbbells sway you. If the presence of hardbodies of either sex is motivating to you, great, but if they are too distracting and cause you to loose focus and keep you from training hard, then its not great. Getting strong is hard work and requires focus and concentration. But if you elect to join a gym it is important that you choose a place that you like and will enjoy going to. Aside from that look for these things:

1) Safety. Ask yourself these questions: Is the place well lit? Clean, including restrooms? Free of accident causing clutter? Are weight plates and dumbbells picked up? Exits and fire exits well marked? Are there first aid kits available and accessible? Is the staff CPR certified? Is the neighborhood safe? Is the parking area well lit? Is the staff willing to accompany lady members to their cars after dark?

2) Equipment. Look for a good selection, preferably both machines and free weights, arranged well, of good quality, and well maintained.

3) Hours. Are they open when you want to work out?

4) Convenience. Is it close enough and easy enough to get to so that using it can become a habit?

5) Crowding. Unfortunately, it is not an uncommon practice for a gym/spa/club to oversell memberships. This is understandable in a business sense, as it is a sales driven industry, but often this results in a crowded facility where you have to always wait to use the equipment, and is noisy, dirty, and under-equipped. Some places even require you to sign a waiting list to use a piece of equipment, then limit your time once it is your turn.

6) Knowledgeable staff. You don't have to have champion bodybuilders on site, but you do need someone there at all times that can show you how to use the equipment safely, give you a spot when you require one, and answer basic training questions.

7) Cost. This is a factor to most people, even for membership at a spartan gym. Some of the larger chains charge an initiation or 'start-up' fee of two hundred (plus) dollars, and a monthly charge of a hundred dollars or more, especially for a couple's or family membership. Other chain 'spas' and 'fitness centers' advertise memberships for "less than twenty dollars a month", but don't disclose in their ads that it's a limited use membership restricted to certain off-peak hours or certain days of the week. These are 'lifetime' memberships that you can only 'upgrade' (for a greater monthly fee) but never cancel. Beware of 'special' prices available "today only", especially an unbelievably good discount for a 'lifetime' membership. Don't bite. 'Lifetime' is defined by the gym and can mean virtually anything. Another chain, well-known in the last few years, charges only ten dollars a month, but will never notify you of changes to this agreement, and will actually bar you from using the facility if you grunt, sweat, breathe hard, or make a noise with a weight. They care only about selling memberships, NOT

providing you with a place to actually work out. Again, *caveat emptor*.

I will readily admit to being spoiled on the subject of cost. I worked and trained for many years at a large gym in Falls Church, Virginia, one of the most well-equipped weight-training facilities on the east coast, but it was not an especially fancy or expensive place. There was over twenty thousand square feet filled with great equipment, some of it quite unique. Based on the cost of a one year membership there, training three times a week worked out to about three dollars per workout. This is a bargain. My membership was free because I worked there, so the cost of my workouts was only sweat.

Gyms sometimes give even part-time employees and subs a free membership. See if a local gym needs someone to work the front desk on an early morning or graveyard shift a day or two a week. You may get to work out for free and make a dollar in the process, plus it is motivating to just be in the gym environment around people that are working out.

ATTIRE

Other things you will need, if not already in possession of them, are proper attire and shoes. Believe me, you don't need the latest spandex outfit and high-tech footwear. This does not impress real gym people, and in fact, can make you the subject of some ribbing. What you do need are comfortable shorts or long sweat pants, a comfortable, loose-fitting t-shirt or muscle tank, and a good pair of athletic shoes. Any good pair of running shoes is adequate, something with decent arch support. If you care to get shoes specifically for weight training, they are available, but be prepared to shell out some bucks. I see some guys lifting in work boots and this seems to work well enough, but don't try to do your cardio in them. Duh.

David and Peter Paul Barbarian used to work out in combat boots, bib overalls, and flannel shirts. They didn't care one bit about spandex or looking like the height of gym fashion. They did bicep curls with a pair of one hundred fifty pound dumbbells and were renowned as powerful squatters as well. These guys came to the gym to **train**.

While you don't need the latest fashion in gym attire, you <u>do</u> need to keep your gym clothes, including footwear, CLEAN and ODOR FREE. I have seen people barred from gyms because they wouldn't launder their workout clothes, and others who should've been. They were oblivious or perhaps just uncaring of the fact that they *stunk*.

CONDUCT

These smelly guys (and there are a few gals who fall into this category as well) are often the same idiots who use foul language in a loud voice, sport t-shirts with obscene words, abuse the equipment, don't pay their dues on time, don't re-rack their weights, and spit on the floor and in the drinking fountains. They think that this is 'hard-core'. Do not be one of these cretins. Show respect and consideration for the other gym members, the facility, and yourself. Good conduct is it's own reward, but it will pay off in tangible ways for you eventually. Consider the following monologue. I paraphrase what I have actually heard ladies say in gyms many times.

"There's this one really strong man at the gym with huge arms and I wanted to ask him about what I should do for triceps. He works out <u>so hard</u> that I was a little nervous to approach him and speak with him, but he turned out to be really nice and was so polite and helpful. He's actually a real gentleman. Oh, I hope he's there again today. I'll ask him about his glutes."

This versus: "There's this big guy at the gym and he must not have washed for months he smells so bad, and he spits and curses and never puts back his weights. He is *so gross* that I just dread going in there anymore. I spoke with the manager and said that if they don't do something about him I'm not going to renew my membership when it's up next week. You should talk to them and tell them the same thing."

Gyms are businesses. If their bottom line suffers because of you a totally legal reason can and will be found to terminate your membership. Trust me.

On the opposite end of the spectrum are the men and women that practically bathe in cologne or perfume. They walk by and a second later you are enveloped in a cloud of scent so heavy you are gasping for breath and your eyes are watering. They do this probably because they are too worried about body odor. Believe me, if your body and your gym clothes are clean you can work up quite a sweat and offend no one with your odor. In fact pheromones, sex hormones, are present in sweat. If you sweat *clean* you might be pleasantly surprised at some of the attention you get.

It would seem like a real no-brainer that you shouldn't work out when you're ill, yet I have seen many, many people come into the gym sick with colds, flu, and worse, and attempt to exercise. There are so many things wrong with this I hardly know where to begin. Most importantly, they are exposing everyone there to whatever it is they have. This is not just inconsiderate, it is almost criminally negligent. Secondly, they are prolonging their illness. Weight training and building muscle takes a lot of your energy and this will cause your immune system to function at less than optimal level.

I've actually told people to go home and go to bed instead of working out, and I usually get a response along the lines of: "But I've been in bed for two days! I can't miss another workout!" Or (you guessed it), "Well I just thought I should come in and work it out."

No, you shouldn't.

Exercise in general strengthens the immune system, but what occurs immediately after a vigorous workout is that it is suppressed for several hours. If it is already struggling to combat an illness, suppressing it is the last thing you should be doing.

"But I've been on medication for the last 48 hours so I'm not infectious" is the other excuse I occasionally hear.

Really? And who told you that? And on further query I've sometimes discovered that the 'medication' is cough syrup or some over the counter cold tablets.

These are signs and symptoms of exercise addiction. If this is you then you need to do some serious self-examination and soul-searching. What is really more important to you, your health and that of all those around you, or missing a workout? And can you imagine a more ludicrous or ironic situation than someone compromising their health to exercise?

OTHER WORKOUT GEAR

Another crucial item is a stop watch. I can hear you now. "What?! I want to weight train, not run a race!" I will explain later but for now just trust me – you need a stopwatch. I buy cheap plastic digital stopwatches at a big chain sporting goods store for about ten bucks. I purchased my last one three years ago and still use it daily. Well worth the investment.

You will need to keep track of your workouts. You do not need a computer program or expensive pre-printed workout log. The ones I've seen generally have lots of headings for stuff you do not need to do for this type of training, and lack many for things that are essential. You do need at least a spiral notebook and something to write with, preferably not crayons or eyeliner.

A pair of straps for your pulling movements is a good idea. There is a type on the market that puts a wide leather flap directly in your palms. Wrapped around a bar and gripped this makes it virtually impossible to loose your grip. They are excellent, though they wear quickly. Metal hook attachments are interesting to use, but Buddy Klemek and I straightened out a pair doing heavy (**heavy!**) shrugs on a standing shrug machine. (A shrug *machine*? Yes, I told you there was some unique equipment in my gym).

There are good straps of cotton webbing and of leather. I use a pair of straps of unique yet old-school design, made from an old military cotton web belt. My cost was zero but for the time to sew the ends together at a right angle and the thread to do it with. You must use COTTON webbing for this. Nylon webbing will slip on the apparatus. These form a closed teardrop shape and are superior to the standard type of straps because with a little practice you can secure each of them around the bar using only the fingers of that hand.

If you prefer not to use straps of any kind that's fine, but realize you won't be able to move as much weight in your pulling movements without them. Your grip will give out before the bigger back and shoulder muscles will. There is some virtue in this however, as the forearm muscles, an often ignored muscle group and location of most of your grip strength, will get a great workout without straps. If you don't do specific lifts for forearms, then forget straps.

I have actually seen people using straps while bench pressing, for tricep pressdowns, and overhead presses. Why, I have no idea. They apparently don't understand that pressing against the bar means you are not pulling on it. In actuality this creates a very dangerous situation. Imagine what would happen if you reached muscle failure and your lift collapsed while you were doing an overhead press and the dumbbells were tightly secured to your wrists with straps? You would be lucky to get away with only a concussion, or a broken collar bone and torn delts. Doing them without straps and failing would be embarrassing when you dropped them on the floor, but at least you could avoid caving your head in or breaking your shoulder. Straps and hooks are wonderful workout aids, but only if used properly.

On lifting belts: If you need one, use one. Due to a minor back condition I require one when I lift heavy, which is most of the time, especially when doing squats and/or other heavy leg movements. This is another item you can spend big bucks on if you are of a mind to, but you really need nothing more than a plain, strong leather or nylon lifting belt that is comfortable and has a good solid buckle. If you do not need one it is probably a good idea to avoid learning to rely on one for anything but squats and deadlifts. However, if you intend

on testing your strength with one rep maximums, <u>use one</u>.
Watch the world's strongest man and woman competitions.
Performing incredible feats of power and muscle endurance is
their life's work. They wear belts. It ain't for fun.

Knee wraps, same thing. If you need them, use them,
but only while actually lifting. Between sets, loosen them up
and avoid constricting and possibly injuring the tendons on
either side of your knees.

Gloves. I like workout gloves but strictly speaking they
are not essential. The right pair can aid your grip somewhat,
pad your hands during pushing and pressing movements, and
they look cool. Chalk used to be *de rigeur* in gyms everywhere
and personally I like to see it used still, for nostalgia's sake if
nothing else, but nothing upsets gym staff and other members
like the messy use of chalk, and a good set of gloves might be a
better choice for this reason. When performing pulling
movements there is no real need for them, especially if using
straps or hook attachments. I have a client that wears her pretty
green fingerless workout gloves at all times in the gym, even on
leg day. She likes them and they help her to mentally get in
gear for her workouts. So be it.

Once common as an alternate to gloves and chalk but
almost never seen anymore is the use of sponges to aid one's
grip and pad the palms. Big, natural sponges, not the little
multicolored ones you use to wash dishes. They do work well
and are relatively inexpensive, although using them does look
rather odd.

One other thing that can be a big help in your workouts
is music. It can motivate and energize you and put you in a
great mood. Most gyms have music playing, though the
selection often leaves a lot to be desired. There are a number of
personal music systems available. It's hard to beat the
convenience and unobtrusiveness of the various types of MP3
players. They are small, wont skip, and with the right
headphones (again, get the best ones you can afford) you'll
forget its even there but for the music in your ears. They can be
pricey though. If you get good radio reception in your gym

those headphones with the little integral AM/FM receivers are excellent in terms of convenience and cost.

Whatever you choose, use it in considerate fashion. The cop on the power bench next to you doesn't want to hear your favorite gangsta rap, and you probably do not want to listen to my selection of Irish sea chanties. Even with headphones on be aware and considerate and keep the volume at the minimum you need to enjoy your music. Oh, and please try to not sing along with it.

Bear in mind that using these wonderful gadgets isolates you from the fit, happy, and energetic people all around you in the gym. Yes, the point of going to the gym is to work out, but it is also a great place to meet people.

Nothing makes those interminable cardio sessions fly by like stimulating conversation with the interesting person next to you. You will meet a better bunch of people in the gym than you will sitting on a barstool, so turn off the music once in awhile and *engage*. 'Nuff said. Okay, lets go.

TRAINING FREQUENCY

TRAIN HARD - BUT DON'T <u>OVER</u>TRAIN

One of the most common mistakes that people make in their quest to get bigger and stronger is overtraining. They start to see positive results and naturally get enthused but then fall victim to a classic mistake, thinking that if three workouts a week are good then six will be twice as good. World-class bodybuilders with artificially enhanced recovery ability might need daily, full-body workouts. The rest of us do not.

Here is the place to disillusion many readers of another commonly held but very wrong notion. You do not build your muscles in the gym. Quite the contrary; you tear them down. This stimulates muscle growth, but the actual growth then occurs only in the recovery phase when you sleep, so if you are short-changing yourself on sleep you are also short-changing yourself on muscle growth. This is a terribly common flaw in many peoples workout regimen.

Many are the times I have been approached, usually – though not always – by twenty-something year old guys and gals with the hopes that I can tell them why they are not making any gains. I first ask all the obvious questions. Are they varying their workouts? Are they challenging themselves? Are they getting adequate protein and eating right? Are they overtraining? Often these young people are dedicated, focused, and possess decent training knowledge and are managing these things properly. Then I ask how much sleep they're getting and a perplexed look comes over them. "Huh? What does **that** have to do with it?"

So I explain the crucial recovery phase and physiological muscle growth occurring only during sleep, and the perplexed look changes to one of rueful realization, sometimes shock. A common excuse then is "But I'm in school and I only sleep about three or four hours a night!" Or something along the lines of "I'm a real night owl. I can't get to bed before three AM 'cause I'm out with my friends." My perhaps too pat reply to this is, "well, it's all a matter of priorities." If partying is your priority then working out can't be, and vice versa.

Weight training causes microscopic muscle tears and when they heal, assimilating protein into themselves, your muscles become larger and stronger. These microtraumas are a cause of the muscle soreness you feel a day or sometimes two after a strenuous workout. They can also be the result of too-vigorous stretching, especially if the individual is not very limber. If these tears are larger than microscopic, then it is an injury, and this is to be avoided at all costs. If the entire muscle or muscle group hurts to some extent it is muscle soreness. If the pain is intense and localized it is probably a tear. If this occurs don't screw around. Ice it and get to a doctor ASAP.

When beginning a vigorous weight training program you **will** experience periods of muscle soreness. These will become less intense as you progress and become conditioned, but everyone that trains hard experiences this from time to time and sometimes it can be quite severe. I typically experience this muscle soreness beginning forty-eight hours after a workout, but it can start as long as ninety-six hours afterwards. It is known as DOMS (Delayed Onset Muscle Soreness) and how long it lasts is a function of nutrition (including water), rest, and your own individual recovery ability.

A deep muscle soreness in a large muscle group like quads can be painful to the point of temporary debilitation, yet not be an injury. I usually start to feel this on the second day after I do heavy squats, and it makes walking and negotiating stairs quite difficult. Curiously, going down stairs becomes more difficult than going up. If your pain is this great there is no need to be stoic. Take an aspirin or some other over the counter pain reliever.

It is also helpful to get on the treadmill or stationary bike and do fifteen or twenty minutes at a medium pace immediately after a heavy leg workout, if you can. It won't keep you from experiencing DOMS altogether, but it can help keep it from being so severe.

It is still commonly believed that lactic acid buildup in the muscles is the cause of muscle soreness. The saying "feel the burn," is meant to refer to that. It is mistakenly thought that this "burn" arises from the searing of the fibers with lactic acid that builds up in them during exercise. I've even seen people drinking bicarbonate of soda before they work out, not because of indigestion but to "neutralize lactic acid". When the muscles demand for energy is high, lactate concentration does begin to rise, but this is a beneficial process that ensures energy production can continue. Excess lactate is removed by the body through oxidation and conversion to glucose. The acidic form of lactate - lactic acid - is NOT produced in the muscles.

And this all leads me to the guiding principle of this section on training frequency. *When training for muscle strength and size there is never any profit in working out a muscle that is still sore from a previous workout.* If you continue to train sore muscles and break them down further before they are fully recovered from a previous workout, the eventual result will be *smaller*, *weaker* muscles, not larger, stronger ones.

So let your body be your guide. For example, if your legs are sore from squats two days ago, it is fine to go to the gym and weight train, *but not your legs.* This concept would seem self-evident, yet I often see people so sore they can barely hold a weight, doing the very same lifts that they did just the day before that caused the soreness.

I'm certain that at least part of the reason for this is that coaches and phys-ed teachers everywhere used to drill into players and students the fact that they had to "work it out" when they felt pain. I am a proponent of many old-school training methods, but not this one. There is no telling how many people have been screwed up for life by this. I'd like to give those old s.o.b.'s a good quad tear and then make them "work it out" on the squat rack or by running laps. Do **not** work it out! Rest it. Let it heal.

As you progress and your muscles become conditioned, the severity of the muscle soreness you feel will decrease, and you will get sore less often, up to a point. A vigorous workout, particularly a leg workout, will still sometimes make my muscles sore, but I love the feeling, when I can achieve it, because I know it means that I had a great workout and then my muscles will grow. It does require me putting a hundred and one percent into my workout though. Remember, the more you improve, the more difficult it becomes to make further improvement. I would say this applies to all facets of life, not just weight training. Gee, philosophy in a weight training manual, who would've thought?

Actually, another really excellent training guide is the Heavy Duty series by the late, great Mike Mentzer, and it does contain his philosophies. I read his books, was privileged to speak with him upon occasion, and train with men who trained with him, and I know that anything he said or wrote on the subject of weight training is well worth paying attention to.

To bring Mike's training methodology into a more contemporary reference, he trained Dorian Yates – a name most afficionados of the muscle/bodybuilding world should be familiar with. Dorian said that his arms grew noticeably as the result of a *single* heavy duty workout Mike put him through, and Dorian's arms were already huge at that time.

Mike's method, very basically, was to train brutally hard, usually using the pre-exhaust method, train briefly (his workouts sometimes lasted less than twenty minutes), and train infrequently, allowing maximum time for recovery. At times he worked out only twice a week. It worked for him. He was the only man to win the Mr. America contest with a *perfect* 300 score, and talk about strong . . . He and his brother Ray trained with weights that would give pause to a power lifter, poundages that only a handful of their contemporaries could even consider. They were strength legends in an arena of very strong men.

INJURIES

Aside from the ache of a good workout there is pain that is indicative of certain types of injuries, and it would behoove you to be aware of these: separations, sprains, strains, and tendinitis. I include this section on injuries in the chapter on training frequency because they all can be symptoms of overtraining.

Strains are probably the most common muscle injury. They are also referred to as pulled muscles. They are in fact tears (larger than the microtrauma of a good workout) in muscle tissue, that can occur suddenly or gradually following prolonged or extreme contractions of muscle (i.e. *weight training*). A mild strain might cause only a dull ache, but when more serious it can result in a sharp, severe pain accompanied by swelling and bruising. In the case of bad tears, particularly when large muscles like quads or pecs are involved, surgery may be required, and the sooner the better. I once saw Jeff Everson (one time editor-in-chief of Muscle and Fitness, and a bodybuilder and weightlifter of some note in his day) at the time of a massive pec tear he experienced. His side from his armpit to his hip was one massive bruise from the blood leakage beneath his skin from his injury. Needless to say he underwent surgery within short order.

Separations happen when the muscle separates from the bone that it is anchored to. These are serious, painful, and relatively rare, thank goodness. Oddly perhaps, I've actually never seen this happen in the gym, but I've seen it occur more than once as the result of an accident.

My friend and role-model Phil Evanisko, an extremely dedicated, focused, and **safe** bodybuilder, once suffered a very serious separation of one of his quadriceps from a fall on ice one winter. Wisely, though I know it was supremely frustrating to him, he did not attempt to work out until he was completely healed and recovered. This took **nine months**. Separations are serious injuries.

Sprains are injuries occurring directly to the ligaments

and/or joints. A sprain most commonly occurs to an ankle, but sometimes to a knee or wrist, or even less commonly an elbow or shoulder, when you turn it accidentally while it is under a load, such as when lifting or running. It will be tender and swollen and will likely bruise. In severe cases they can actually be more painful than a broken bone and take longer to heal.

Tendinitis can also be quite painful. This occurs when the tendon becomes inflamed, usually from prolonged overuse, but sometimes from a trauma or the improper use of lifting wraps. In chronic cases the body, in an effort to protect the tendon, will deposit a calcium layer in the joint which in turn can cause arthritis and/or a bone spur. In the gym it most commonly (though an uncommon condition itself) is the result of performing heavy wrist curls, leg curls, or improper positioning while doing leg extensions. I am not an advocate of leg extensions and don't normally recommend doing them at all, for this and other reasons I'll address later.

Something virtually identical to tendinitis occurs as the result of bearing a light muscular load in a repetitive motion over a long period of time and is known as carpal tunnel syndrome.

I once suffered tendinitis so bad that when I pressed my ear to my forearm and clenched and unclenched my fists, I could *hear* the tendons grating back and forth. Ironically, this was not a result of anything I did in the gym, but from *trimming hedges* all day with a big manual clipper. I theorize that the unnatural hand position this forced me to assume for a prolonged time constricted the carpal tunnels and the impact of the blades clacking together for several hours traumatized the same spot on the tendons repeatedly. That this was continued in the face of steadily increasing discomfort was due to a separate condition I sometimes suffer from called cranial-anal displacement.

When your body adapts and periods of muscle soreness become less frequent and less severe it is then time to get on a very regular schedule of training. A Monday, Wednesday, Friday schedule seems to be the one people like to use the most, probably because it makes good sense in terms of most people's schedules and is easy to remember. Of course it can actually be any three days with every-other-day frequency, for approximately your first year of weight training.

Generally, after your first year following this cycle of training you will no longer be a beginning weight trainer. You will have moved on to the intermediate level and will perhaps need or want to train more frequently. The logical modification to your cycle then is to begin to run through it on three consecutive days, Monday, Tuesday, and Wednesday for example, then repeat the cycle again on Thursday, Friday, and Saturday. Rest Sunday. Notice that this still allows your bodyparts seventy-two hours rest before training them again. But it does double your training volume, and this may be too much when first entering this intermediate phase. If in fact this places too much demand on your time, energy, and recovery ability, then a more reserved increase is in order, as follows:

Continue your Monday, Wednesday, Friday cycle, then on Saturday begin to repeat the cycle. Note that then the final workout of your cycle will occur that next Wednesday rather than Friday, and you will no longer always be doing the same workout on the same day of the week because your schedule is no longer static - it begins to cycle. If and when you become able to take on more, then add Tuesday to the cycle. If and when, etc. add Thursday to the cycle. Keep Sunday a rest day. This day of not working out is important in your quest to become stronger, and I'd go so far as to say that on that day you should try to not do anything too physically demanding. Mowing the yard is probably fine. Moving your brother-in-law's piano up three flights is not.

This intermediate status will be for a lengthier time than the one year spent as a beginner. In fact it may last forever. Many people never progress beyond it for many different reasons, most commonly because they have no need or desire to, and there is nothing wrong with this. This level of training will result in a higher degree of fitness and strength than most people ever obtain, and it still takes up only six to seven hours per week.

Someone with a few years of this intermediate level of cycled training under their belt may go on to an advanced level wherein the cycle is repeated in the same order but performing two of the divisions within the same visit to the gym, or at least on the same day, meaning two visits to the gym that day. This brings us nicely to the next section.

TRAINING DIVISIONS

A beginners triple-split routine, based on a Monday, Wednesday, Friday schedule is as follows:

Monday.   Legs and abs.
Wednesday. Back and biceps.
Friday.   Chest and triceps.

Now, it really doesn't matter what order you start these in. Back and biceps on Monday would be perfectly fine for example, but whatever order you start them in, it is important that you *keep them in that same order,* so that you never train the same muscle groups on any two consecutive workout days. This way there is adequate time for rest and recuperation, i.e. muscle growth. On this type of routine it is okay to do a low intensity cardio and stretching workout on the alternate days. In fact this would only benefit your weight training, if not done to excess.

I know what some of you are thinking right now. "What?! This is only one workout a week per muscle group!"

The answer to this: Yep.

Monday. Legs and abs.

Because our Monday workout is a leg workout and these muscles are the largest we have, it involves heavy weights to stimulate muscle growth, but heavy is a relative term. Your definition of heavy may not be the same as my definition of heavy. There is a very specific but individual definition of heavy as it applies to cycled training, and this addressed and defined in the section on training cycles. This is a good place to relate this bit of training advice. Do your heaviest lifts first when you are freshest and have the most energy. This applies to all workouts, not just legs.

People are often surprised to learn how few different lifts are required for a complete leg workout. There are but three essential movements. Yes, yes. I can hear the hue and cry now. Bear with me. You bought this manual in hopes that it contained something different, didn't you? Contempt prior to investigation is a practice that will always keep you from learning anything.

LEG PRESS. This is the most basic of basics. In the beginning your leg workout should start with these. There are great alternatives to this and we'll address these in a moment, but in the beginning use this movement. Leg presses are done for the quadriceps, that is, the front of the upper legs. Secondarily they involve the glutes, or butt muscles, quite strongly also if done with your feet toward the top of the foot plate and bringing the knees as close to your face as safely possible. Regardless of where you place your feet they should always be angled so that your toes are slightly outward. This will allow natural motion of the knee joint.

I realize that some people may have knee problems that preclude doing these except with an abbreviated range of motion. They will need to do something else for the butt, perhaps straight-legged deadlifts. These should be done by a beginner only under supervision and with conservative weight.

The minimum range of motion for a normal leg press is from starting with your upper and lower legs at a right angle and then pressing out to almost, but not quite, full extension. That is, press out until your legs are just shy of lockout. Locking out on this lift is hard on your knees and it allows you to rest, which is not what you want to do at this point. Remember you are trying to fatigue the muscle and anything that allows you to rest is not helping to do this. Rest between sets, not between reps.

If you are limber enough and have no knee problems, try to start the movement with your knees at less than a right angle, that is, with your knees closer to your face. The right angle rule is the *minimum* for a good leg press.

There is an interesting variation of the standard leg press called the plie` press, in which you place your feet with the toes at an extreme outward angle. You will have to lessen the weight to perform these properly, but they affect the quads and glutes in quite a different fashion and are worth doing once in awhile.

The alternatives for leg presses are the various types of squats and lunges. Experienced lifters can do squats with a barbell off the squat rack. Those less experienced should do them on a Smith machine. If one of these excellent pieces of equipment are not available, then body weight squats also known as deep knee bends, are okay to start. If these are not challenging enough for you, then try doing them while holding a pair of dumbbells straight down at your sides, or one-legged while stabilizing yourself with one hand.

Remember, with squats you must move the weight of your body in addition to whatever extra weight you have selected. I have frequently fielded questions along the lines of "What's wrong with my squat? I can leg press four hundred pounds but can only squat two hundred." To which I inquire how much they weigh and they'll say, (you guessed it) "about two hundred pounds. Why?"

Of course we don't include our bodyweight in the figure when talking about how much we squat, but actually that is what we do. When these folks are told that basically they *have* squatted with four hundred pounds, that is, two hundred pounds of weights plus two hundred pounds of bodyweight, you can practically see the light bulb come on over their heads.

There are several variations of lunges and they are good to great quad and glute exercises. Walking lunges are performed by stepping out with a longer than normal stride and bending the knees until the knee of the trailing leg is only a couple inches off the floor. Shove off immediately and step out again as soon as fully upright. For added intensity hold dumbbells in your hands. I've seen people doing these and the other types of lunges with a barbell across their shoulders but I can't recommend this. It places too much weight up too high and because you are traveling while doing them this makes stability a problem. It also causes you to take up too wide a swath of the gym floor thus creating not only a hazard to yourself but to your fellow gym members as well. Safety first. Always.

Stationary lunges make you less of a nuisance and spectacle to others. These are done by lunging out, as with walking lunges, but then keeping your feet planted in that position and doing a set of what are essentially squats in a stride position. Three sets of ten for one leg then the other, or you can alternate sides, set to set. When you get good at these try them while holding dumbbells. The other great way to do these is on a Smith machine, with added weight or no.

Finally, the most difficult, so not surprisingly, the most effective way to perform lunges is to do what used to be called California Lunges. These are begun in a manner identical to the stationary lunges but when you rise up at the end of the rep you give an extra push, bringing the front leg back and placing that foot back beside the other to achieve a normal stance. The front foot is up off the ground in this last part of the movement and this puts extra stress on the hamstrings and glutes of the other leg. Again, for added intensity hold dumbbells in your hands. If you've never done lunges do not start with these. Work your way up to this variation, getting a feel for the movement and developing your balance as you do. If you have problems with your balance avoid them altogether and stick with the stationary type.

Lets address the subject of leg extensions as I promised earlier. They are a very common movement for the quads. In fact, they are much too common. I see many people who do no other leg movement but extensions, much to their detriment. Leg extensions place you in a weaker position to exercise your quads than do leg presses, or actually any of the other lifts mentioned above, and they tend to be hard on your knees as well. Of course lifting a great amount of weight is not the actual aim with this type of training, building functional strength is – and there is a difference. If you are going to perform them, avoid knee trauma by adjusting the seat of the machine so that there is approximately a finger-width space between the back of your knee and the edge of the seat.

If, like most people when they do these, your seat position is so far back that the back of your knee is tight against the edge of the seat, you will constrict the free movement of the big tendons located there, and quite possibly injure them over time. On the other hand, do not have your knee several inches from the seat edge. You need more support than that in this movement that already places your knees in a weak position. With these provisions in mind, if you have the time, energy, and desire to do leg extensions go right ahead, but only *in addition to* leg presses, never *instead of* them.

LEG CURLS. These are for the hamstrings, or the back of the upper legs. Secondarily these also work the glutes, or butt. They're hard, and I know very few people that actually like doing them. It is an unnatural way to lift a weight, and has an awkward feel because of this, but for hamstring development they are crucial. There are different types of leg curl apparatus available, the best being the prone, two-legged leg curl machine, and of these, those that put you in a butt-high position are superior to those that are simply flat. There is also an important safety consideration for this movement, similar to that for leg extensions. When doing leg curls on a prone machine, your kneecap should *not* be on the platform, and there should *never* be more than a finger-width space between the top of your kneecap and the edge of the pad. These finger width rules are important and easy to remember and your measuring device is always handy. Heed them. The movement should be a controlled one from full extension of the legs to actually just touching your glutes with the roller pads, then back down to full extension. There are usually handles underneath to grasp onto – use them. Make sure your chest is in full, tight contact with the pad at all times – NO arching of the back. This will lead to a lower back injury.

The seated, two-legged leg curl machine is also a good

one, providing a good, secure base for the lower back, but placing you in a weaker position to actually perform the movement. In the interest of safety its an acceptable trade-off.

There are also one-legged leg curl machines. I don't think much of them. With some you stand to perform the movement, with others you crouch, with your weight resting on your knees and forearms. These are generally considered machines for 'shaping' and 'finishing' the hamstrings, rather than for actual strength building. Even the best of these put you in an awkward and unbalanced position to perform a leg curl, and can easily cause you to injure your lower back.

An interesting and effective alternate to the leg curl is the stiff-legged deadlift, and it is especially effective when combined with a back movement - back hyperextensions, because of the strong involvement of the glutes in both. If you're able, you could do these occasionally just for variety. But they also involve the muscles of the lower back and if you, like many people, suffer from pain in the lower lumbar area, my advice is that you should not attempt them. Like any lift they are perfectly safe if performed perfectly, but frankly, the chances for injury while doing these are greater than most other lifts. For this reason I also don't recommend them for beginners and so, while they are an effective hamstring exercise, I won't outline them here. When you become an intermediate lifter, probably after your first year or so of diligent training, and want to try stiff-legged deads, please research them thoroughly and seek out the guidance of a trainer or other experienced lifter. For now stick with leg curls.

CALF RAISES. These are done for the calves. Duh. It is possible to build enormous strength in your calves. Though much smaller, it is possible to train them so they can move far more weight than even your biggest muscle group, your quads. Reg Park, Arnold Schwarzenegger's idol, was capable of calf raises with nearly a thousand pounds. Reg was obviously a very strong guy but I guarantee you he didn't squat with that much.

I am blessed with good calves. They are a particularly

strong bodypart for me. I occasionally do sets of fifteen reps with nine hundred forty pounds on a donkey calf raise machine, though my usual workout weight is usually eight hundred fifty. This is a relatively rare piece of equipment, but it is absolutely superb for building strength and muscle mass in the calves. Obviously, it places you in a very powerful position to work your calves. Unless you are fortunate enough to have access to one of these unique machines, you're stuck doing donkey calf raises the old fashioned way: With your feet flat on the floor, bend forward at the waist and place your forearms firmly on a bench. Have your training partner or some other willing participant sit on your back, straddling your hips. Raise up on your tiptoes as far as possible, then lower slowly until your feet are flat on the floor again. It looks odd, yes, but it is an excellent movement for calves. When you become used to this movement you then graduate to performing them with just the balls of your feet and toes on the edge of a low platform or two by four. This is much superior and is the way they really should be done because you can then let your heels down lower than your toes at the bottom of the movement, thus performing them over a greater range of motion.

I have seen men do donkey calf raises with more than one person on their backs. There is a fairly famous picture taken by Art Zeller of Arnold doing these with Franco Columbu, Frank Zane, and another unidentified fellow perched on him. Early in his career calves were a weak bodypart for Arnold and because of this he did most of his posing for photographs while standing in water. Then at one point they seemed to just appear overnight miraculously. I wonder if this movement had something to do with it.

The other perfectly acceptable and less unusual-looking movement for calves is the standing calf raise. Any good gym will have at least one of these machines. Be certain that you keep your hips, back, and shoulders in a straight line while doing these, and that the height adjustment is set so as to allow you a full range of motion, both up and down, without topping out or bottoming out the machine. If no such machine is available they can be done on the edge of a stable platform while holding a dumbbell in one hand and hanging on to something immobile with your other hand. To add intensity they can be done on one leg.

I can't use the standing calf raise machine to any great effect because my calves are exceptionally strong and with the weight required to give them even an adequate workout the pads cause severe bruising on the top of my trapezius muscles. However, it is a standard in gyms and is fine as a muscle builder for most people.

Calf raises can also be done on any leg press machine. Just place your feet so that only your toes and the ball of your foot is on the platform and do the raises the regular way. If the machine has safety stops, use them for this movement.

The other thing you will have to do sometimes for calves is a seated calf raise. These machines are less common than standing calf raise machines but again, well-equipped gyms have them. They are occasionally necessary to fully work the soleus muscle, say every third leg workout, instead of one of the others.

With these three basic exercises, leg press, leg curl, and calf raise, you've worked all your leg muscles. This is why we do abs on leg day. There is lots of time to include them in this workout, and not on the other two, if you want to keep your Wednesday and Friday workouts under forty-five minutes.

But what about hack squats? What about those other favorites, the thigh abductor and adductor machines?

I will state that these days hack squats are often the basis of my own leg workout, but I am not a beginner. They are fine muscle builders, but they can cause something called shear stress on the knee joint and are to be avoided by those prone to knee problems. They have not caused me knee problems, and I go heavy when I do them, but then I have never had knee problems. If your knees are in fine shape, and you're are fortunate enough to have a hack machine in your gym, I encourage you to try them, if/when you feel the need to do something for quads other than the leg press. At first, start with

no weight on the apparatus, and experiment with your stance on the foot platform. Be conservative about how quickly and how far you go down on the rack once the apparatus is off the safety stops. If you feel **any** pain in your knees cease immediately and realize that hack squats are not for you. Safety, safety, safety.

HIP/THIGH ABDUCTORS/ADDUCTORS. I include these provisionally. The thigh abductor and adductor muscles are part of your quads and if you've challenged yourself with a good heavy set of leg presses you've already exercised these muscles. If you want to emphasize the development of your inner and outer quads, and have the time and energy to include them, by all means do these two machines. Strictly speaking though, they are not essential. Abductors do also work the glutes strongly, so I occasionally do them for this reason. If one has a knee condition that precludes going knees-to-face in the leg press then these are fine to do *in addition to*, but not instead of the leg press done to the right angle position. If one cannot do straight-legged deadlifts for the glutes, then these are a fair alternative.

Watch who does the abductor and adductor machines. The majority of the people using them are ladies. Chat one of them up sometime and ask them why they do these two movements. Most of the time the answer will be "to make my thighs thinner." Makes me want to scream. *Weight training will not make bodyparts shrink.* If nothing is done about the layer of fat on top of their thighs (that is, doing lots of cardio/aerobics, proper diet and nutrition) and they persist in weight training them and building up the muscle, the end result will be LARGER thighs, not smaller. Many people are also under the impression that doing lots of ab movements will give them a narrow waist and they are wrong for the exact same reason. I repeat: weight training, especially *this* type of weight training, causes your muscles to grow, not to shrink! Do you ever see anyone doing barbell curls to make their biceps smaller? Bench presses to shrink their chest?

ABS. Many people feel it is fine to do abs every day. Terise Anderson, an accomplished trainer at my gym, adheres to this, and I can't argue with her success. She was a successful pro bodybuilder with the trophies in her office to prove it. She is one of the stronger ladies you will ever meet and has a great set of abs. Gorgeous too, and very womanly, disproving again the notion that muscles are unfeminine. Many people do a very high rep, low weight or unweighted ab routine and some actually get some results this way. I have a friend, a great guy though 'somewhat' stubborn, who does a minimum of one hundred fifty reps for abs with moderate weight on a particular ab machine five days a week. After two solid years of this he is starting to see his six pack.

It is possible for some people to develop incredible stamina in this muscle group. Three time Mr. Olympia Frank Zane once did situps on a Roman chair for <u>two and a half hours,</u> nonstop, at a steady pace. 'Zabo' Kozewski used to do one thousand situps *as a warmup*.

For me personally, doing a high-rep ab workout every day never worked very well in developing their size. They only began to become really noticeable when I started working them with the cycled training method, that is once a week, hard, with weighted movements. If this just isn't enough for you, then I suggest that you add an unweighted ab movement to your Wednesday and/or Friday workouts.

My favorite calisthenic, or unweighted movement for abs is ab circles. Perform them like this: On a simple angled ab bench seat yourself securely with feet firmly beneath the rollers, and recline to a forty-five degree angle. Cross your hands over your chest and describe a circle with your torso. One full revolution is one rep. Do ten clockwise reps then, without stopping, do ten counter-clockwise reps. This is one set. Do three sets. You may vary the geometry of this movement from workout to workout by elongating the circle into an oval, or by holding yourself at less than, or more than, a forty-five degree angle.

Another simple and effective movement for abs is the

old-fashioned ab wheel. These are still available and they still work. Good for lower back too. Just remember to hold your back with a slight convex curve throughout the motion. Don't allow yourself to become swaybacked while performing these. If you can't do this you're better off leaving them alone.

Generally, for the purposes of this triple-split power cycle, its best to train abs on a weight machine as outlined here, just once a week, at the end of your leg workout.

Your gym will likely have a few different machines where you can work your abs with weighted movements. Most of these focus on upper abs and this is fine if you also then include something like hanging leg raises for your lower abs and hip flexors. The best overall ab machines in my experience are the old-style duo-ab machines. These are the 'folding' machines, that is, hinged in the middle, causing you to have to pull from both ends, i.e. with hands and feet, thus working your upper and lower abs simultaneously, along with your hip flexors. Most commonly these are seated machines, but there are good ones in which you lie on your back and 'fold'.

If you are not fortunate enough to have something like this available, then look for a spot where you can lie on a high bench and grasp something immobile above your head with both hands. A pillar or the end of the bench will do. With your lower legs together but hanging loosely straight down off the edge of the bench, bend at the hips and raise your knees towards your elbows. When you are bent at the waist as far as you can, curl your lower back up and lift your hips and tailbone off the bench. Touch your knees to your elbows and then slowly, in controlled fashion, lower your legs back down until you are once more lying flat with your legs hanging down off the end from the knees down. This is one rep. Repeat.

DO NOT straighten out your legs and use their weight and momentum to throw them up over your head. Not only is this poor form and will not benefit you much, it can lead to injury. Bend your knees and keep your upper calves in contact with your lower hamstrings through all but the very beginning and end of the movement when your lower legs should be dangling off the end of the bench.

When these are no longer so difficult, you can further challenge yourself by finding a bench or platform on which you can perform them at a heads-up angle. An angle with your head even four inches higher than your hips can cause these to become impossible, so be conservative when raising the angle.

OBLIQUES. There are rotary torso machines to target the obliques. I don't much care for them because their range of motion is greater than what you should try to do. Trying to twist to the full range of motion that these machines are capable of can easily injure your lower back, plus if you build up the obliques by doing lots of weight with these or dumbbell side bends you'll thicken your waistline. Far better are twisting crunches. Left elbow to right knee and vice-versa. Also side sit ups. These work the obliques but tend to not build up their size as much as some of the weighted movements. If you already have a six-pack, try these exercises. If not, focus on the first ab movements in this section and be patient. The obliques are small and will receive some stimulus as assisting muscles in the exercises for the rectus abdominis. For most, abs are one of the most stubborn muscle groups and sometimes take literally years to come in. They can actually be strong and well-developed but not visible because they are obscured by a layer of fat. This is an *extremely* common situation, usually with guys who think that endless sets of crunches are supposed to give them a six-pack, but who wouldn't be caught dead on a treadmill.

When asked what I recommend to bring out the abs, that is, to make them visible, I tell people to do push-aways. You do these by placing your hands on the edge of the dinner table and pushing yourself away from it. The nice part about these is that one rep is all that is required, but repeat as necessary and perform them daily. Seriously, to make your abs *visible* the main things, even more important than weight training them, are cardio and diet, cardio and diet, cardio and diet.

Wednesday. Back and biceps.

Next is a back and biceps workout. A simple way to think of this is as a pulling workout. All the lifts done on this day are pulling motions of some sort.

COMPOUND BACK ROWS. First in this workout, following the heaviest lift first rule, are usually rows. Done as described, these affect all the muscles of the back to an extent, including the anterior deltoids (back of the shoulder) hence the name compound.   They give depth and thickness to the muscles of the back including the latisimus dorsi, but other movements are necessary to develop the width of these, the largest muscles in the upper body.

For strength and muscle building cable rows are somewhat superior to the type of rowing machines in which you place your chest against a pad and hold your torso still. For rows I generally recommend narrow or medium-width handles, but wide ones are great to use once in awhile. Your legs should be almost but not quite straight, *a la* the extended position in the leg press. Lean forward from the waist and grasp the handle firmly. Lifting straps help here. The whole first part of the motion comes only from shrugging the shoulders straight back. This particular lift is actually easier to do properly with a heavy weight, because this pulls your shoulders forward into a good starting position. With practice you should be able to raise the weight stack a good six to eight inches simply with this shrugging motion. As you shrug back, try to imagine pinching a penny between your shoulder blades and draw them together. When you can't draw them together any further then bend your elbows, bringing the upper arms just past the sides of your body, while you lean back a bit. To involve the lower back get a *little* bit of a backward/forward leaning motion going when doing rows, say twenty degrees backward, then lean forward about the same twenty degrees, letting your arms and shoulders be pulled forward in a controlled fashion. Do not quite set the weight stack down. Repeat.

The hard part for many people is putting this all together in a natural, smooth motion. It will come with practice. Just imagine yourself in a rowboat, propelling yourself across a lake.

LAT PULLDOWNS. Next is a movement to specifically target the lats. Pulldowns help give them width and that beautiful V taper to your back. There are several different types of machines for this movement, but none of them offer any advantage over the basic cable pulldown machine.

You'll still see folks doing pulldowns and presses behind the neck. Don't. Some can do these and it never seems to bother them but in many it causes a painful condition known as an impingement. If you continue to do pulldowns or presses behind the neck in spite of this pain, a rotator cuff tear can result. The way to avoid it is easy. Just do them to the front.

Lean slightly backwards from the waist with a straight spine. Try not to arc your back. For safety, raise your chin slightly so you can watch the bar coming down. Your choice of grip can make a difference. The standard wide overhand grip is good and you should do them this way sometimes, but an underhand grip with hands only slightly wider than shoulder width is better. In this position you can draw your elbows further back, performing the movement through a wider range of motion. It also puts you in a more powerful position so you can actually do a little more weight this way, in spite of the fact that it's a wider range of motion. With most movements the reverse is true.

A great alternative is wide-grip chins, or pull ups. It is not absolutely necessary to perform them so that you actually place your chin over the bar. A wide overhand grip is great for these, and a narrower underhand grip should be used sometimes to hit the lats in a different manner. I train with a former Mr. America who swears by these and he has a *superb* set of lats.

SHRUGS. Trapezius muscles are best worked with what is the simplest and shortest motion in weight training: shrugs. Shrugs are exactly what they sound like. You grasp a dumbbell in each hand and let them hang naturally down at your sides. Stand with a narrow stance and a straight back and shrug your shoulders straight up as far as you can. Lower them slowly and under control. Repeat. Do not let the weight pull your shoulders down quickly and do not round the motion off, either to the front or the back. Do not bend your elbows. Do not bend your knees or flex your hips to give a little bounce to cheat the weight up. Shrug straight up and down.

Strong traps are extremely important. They can save you from a neck injury, or even a broken neck. Not to mention that when a guy has well developed traps it makes him look big. Do shrugs.

I do not usually recommend that other standard for traps, upright rows. It can bring on a condition similar to the impingement caused by doing pulldowns and presses behind the neck. Again, some people will never be bothered by this, but since shrugs are such an effective and safe movement, why risk it as a beginning weight trainer? Do shrugs.

I'm convinced that the trapezius can be the strongest muscles on the body. I worked traps with Buddy Klemek on a shrug machine with an amount of weight that you wouldn't believe. Suffice to say we took turns shrugging the whole weight stack plus every forty-five pound plate the horns on the sides of the machine would hold, plus more on the handles, leaving just enough room to grip them safely.

This was when Buddy straightened out his steel hook attachments. He is a lean and muscular one hundred ninety pounder, a good-sized though not huge man, but he has weight trained very consistently for over twenty-five years and is just exceptionally strong, possessing what is known as muscle maturity. He has no equal on this particular machine, though Ed Cotter, a massive two hundred sixty pound bodybuilder with traps the size of bricks, comes close. I kept up with Buddy until the addition of the final plate, then once I lifted the apparatus my range of motion became very limited and can't really be counted as good reps. I have to work on this one. The point is, do shrugs.

Aw, c'mon Todd, how much was it? A lot. A <u>whole</u>

lot. The machine had an integral weight stack of four hundred pounds that we **far** exceeded by adding plates. To qualify though, this particular standing shrug machine, while a unique and excellent piece of equipment, is not the equivalent of dumbbell shrugs. These are the standard for this movement and should be used primarily. My regular trapezius training is strict shrugs with a pair of one hundred forty pound dumbbells, though I will go heavier occasionally, when I can find heavier. I also get a tremendous forearm workout from this because this kind of weight necessitates gripping the dumbbells so hard. However, I <u>strongly</u> recommend the use of some sort of straps or other grip aid for these. In fact, it is probably impossible for most people, even those with an exceptionally strong grip, to get a good workout for their traps *without* using straps.

LOWER BACK MOVEMENTS. Like traps, the lower lumbar muscles are an extremely important muscle group to develop, for health and safety reasons alone, aesthetics aside. Strong lower back muscles will protect the vulnerable lower spine - location and source of most back trouble.

Even if you already have a lower back condition you <u>can</u> exercise this area if you proceed carefully, using strict form, conservative weights, and limit your range of motion, especially at first. Strengthening these muscles will allow them to take some of the load of your bodyweight up off your lower vertebra, and over time it is possible to develop great strength in them regardless. I speak from experience. I go extremely heavy in many of my back movements yet I have had a lower back condition (a very mild case of scoliosis from an injury) since a young teen. I have trained it with care and diligence for many years to be able to do this. *Proper* exercising of these muscles is excellent for the pain and debility of a back condition. Regardless, when doing lower back movements, everyone should start conservatively and progress in modest steps.

There are several different lower back machines. Some of them are excellent. Some are not. The simplest and best place to start training your lower back is with lower back raises, more commonly called back hyperextensions, but this is a misnomer. Believe me, the very last thing you want to do is hyperextend your lower back. If you don't currently suffer from lower back pain, you very well may if you hyperextend it. The apparatus used for these is commonly called a Roman Chair. To perform these safely you must be positioned so that your hipbones are a good four inches off the front of the pad. Hang straight down from the waist so that your upper body and lower body are at right angles to each other. Raise your upper body until it is **parallel** to the floor. Have someone hold their hand to stop you from lifting above this point until you have a good idea of how far to raise yourself yet not hyperextend. At this point your entire body should be in a straight line. Lower at a moderate rate, under control.

After a time you may start holding a small weight disc, no more than a ten pounder to start, to your chest as you perform these. For safety and comfort don't hold it behind your head. After you progress to become an intermediate weight trainer you may try raising your upper body **very** slightly past parallel with the floor. <u>Never more than an inch or two.</u> Again, have someone hold their hand to stop you from going further than that.

Straight-legged deadlifts, spoken about briefly before in the section on hamstrings, are also excellent strength builders for the lower back, but unless perfect form is observed the chance of incurring injury is too great for a novice. If you must try straight-legged deads, seek out a knowledgeable trainer to teach you proper form and technique and to closely monitor you while you learn to do them properly. This is a lift in which it is crucial that you check your ego at the door and begin with a light weight.

I'll be very frank. At two hundred twenty pounds of bodyweight, when I began performing these I did them with an *empty bar*, under the tutelage of Phil Evanisko, the most knowledgable trainer I know, and was glad I did. If you currently have no back condition and are mature enough to begin performing them with an extremely conservative weight, by all means give them a try. If not, leave them alone. I must admit however that they do build strength and mass.

Good mornings are an old-school move that many may not have even heard of – and this is a good thing, as they carry an even greater risk of lower back injury. I mention them here mainly because my idol and inspiration, the great Paul Anderson was a huge proponent of them. Basically you get into a squat position with a barbell across your shoulders, but instead of squatting you bend forward at the waist into a bow, then back up to the starting position. Bruce Randall was the undisputed king of this lift and his fine and basic text "The Barbell Method to Strength and Fitness" has good explanation and illustration of this lift. Needless to say these are an advanced movement.

Back hypers, done as I described, are **much** safer than good mornings or even straight-legged deadlifts and produce a fine strengthening effect when performed as a part of cycled training.

To see an incredibly developed lower back, find a back shot of Samir Bannout. At the 1983 Mr. Olympia the crowd was agog when he went into his back poses. His lower back muscles stood out individually like little fingers all fanned out. Folks just hadn't seen this before and it was a big factor in his winning this prestigious competition that year. It spawned the term 'Christmas tree', now in common parlance to describe a set of hyper-developed lower back muscles.

PULLOVERS. Pullovers also work the lats strongly and so are rather redundant, as we have at this point already performed lat pulldowns. However they are such an excellent exercise for general upper body strength that if you have time and energy you should definitely include them, at the very least as an alternate to pulldowns. Besides, the lats are the biggest muscle in the upper body and can usually stand another exercise. Pullovers can be done on one of the excellent pullover machines available, or with a flat bench and a dumbbell. With machine pullovers be very careful on the negative portion, when your arms are rotating upwards in front of you and the weights are being lowered. You can go too far up and back on this portion and hurt your shoulders. The guide here is that you should go far enough to feel a stretch in your shoulders, but never any pain. Bring the bar far enough down in the front to actually touch it to your body gently. Do not slam it into yourself. Control, control, control.

The perfectly fine alternative is with a dumbbell and a low flat bench. Lie flat on the bench with your head just off the end of the bench and place a dumbbell on the floor a foot to eighteen inches beyond this end of the bench. Cup both hands under one head of the dumbbell and lift it up over your head, extending your arms out fully, then smoothly arc it down and touch it gently to your solar plexus, then lift it up and over in a smooth return arc over your head. Touch the floor with it gently and repeat.

This is a safer version of the more common way in which you lay on the bench sideways with only your shoulders and upper back supported by it. You and the bench form a T. The rest of the lift is performed the same. This can be a big strain on the lower back and I don't usually recommend doing them in this manner for that reason. If you never experience lower back pain they're probably fine for you to try.

CURLS. There are more ways to do bicep curls than any other lift. Two of the best using dumbbells are incline bench curls and concentration curls. Another excellent curl using a barbell are that old time standard, twenty-ones.

Incline bench curls are NOT 'preacher' curls. They require an adjustable incline bench ("No kidding?") and the use of dumbbells. The greater the angle (that is, the less the angled part of the bench is elevated), the more difficult the curl is because the larger the arc you must curl the weight through, from straight down to up touching the front of the shoulder. The ultimate expression of an incline bench curl is to do them completely prone on a high flat bench, curling the weights through a full three-quarters of a circle. You MUST work up to these, in strength, but even more importantly in the flexibility of your shoulder joint. It is recommended that females or anyone with wide hips do angle bench curls hammer style, that is with the dumbbells held in your hands with palms facing in toward the body throughout the movement, as opposed to holding them with your palms facing forward. This helps you avoid bumping your hips as you perform the curl.

There is a non-traditional technique, based on the old Zottman curl, that can be used when performing these, if you are prepared for some serious effort and muscle burn. They are best done seated. Start the movement hammer style, making absolutely certain to not move your upper arm <u>at all</u>. Your elbows must not lift up and forward, even a fraction of an inch. Once you have lifted the dumbbells up so that your upper and lower arms are at a right angle pause for just an instant and supinate your forearms all the way. That is, twist them completely so that your hands and the dumbbells rotate from a palms-in attitude to palms-up. Curl them up the rest of the way, again without moving the elbows at all, and it probably won't be far, and it will probably hurt. Lower to the right angle position, pause for a moment, pronate back to the palms-in position and lower the rest of the way. Repeat. You will have to use maybe half the weight you normally do in a regular angle bench curl. In fact, the first time I performed these I used half the weight and could do only slightly more than half the number of reps I usually do. These are **hard**. If they are not, then you are lifting your elbows.

I credit Nick Masick with teaching me these. Nick is a huge young man and if it builds size and/or strength he incorporates it his workouts. He is all natural and one of the more knowledgeable and focused young bodybuilders I've ever known, yet he is a modest, pleasant, balanced, well-rounded individual. He is a pleasure to know and to watch train. I do not hesitate to point him out as a role model to other young bodybuilders.

Concentration curls are most often done seated, usually at the very end of a flat bench, with your legs in a wide vee. Grasp a dumbbell in one hand, bend over slightly and butt the elbow of that hand on the inside of that thigh. Let the arm hang straight down and then curl the dumbbell up until you touch the shoulder with it. Lower and repeat.

Twenty-ones are also tough and they can light your arms <u>up</u>. Grasp a barbell or better yet an easy curl bar loaded with something like three quarters of your max ten rep weight. Let it hang straight down and raise it up as if doing a regular curl but stop halfway up. Lower and repeat seven times. Then without stopping raise it all the way up then lower it like a regular curl, but stop halfway down. Raise and repeat seven times. Then without stopping, perform seven regular, full curls. This is ONE set. I have my clients do this entire thing for three sets and they generally can't finish without assistance.   It would be far too much to do all of these movements as part of your bicep workout. Choose one, then do the following.

REVERSE CURLS. This is a 'finishing' movement for your biceps but it strongly involves the top of the forearm, an often ignored muscle. It is simply a curl done with a palms down grip versus the palms up grip of a standard curl. They can be done with anything you use for regular curls, but work particularly well when performed on a preacher curl machine.

FOREARM OR WRIST CURLS. These are for the bottom, or belly, of the forearms. The simplest and best way is to simply let your hand and an inch or two of wrist hang, palm up, over the end of a flat bench and place a dumbbell in it. Bend the wrist all the way forward and up, then let it all the way down, uncurling the fingers as you do so. Repeat. Be careful not to uncurl your fingers too far and drop the dumbbell. Do not lift your' elbow from the bench.

REVERSE WRIST CURLS. These are for the top of the forearm and if you do reverse curls as outlined above you can forego these, but it is a good idea to alternate for variety. Holding a dumbbell, let your hand and an inch of wrist hang over the end of a flat bench, palm down. Bend the wrist all the way back and up, then let it all the way down. Repeat. Do not try to uncurl your fingers on this one – you will drop the weight.

Friday. Chest and Triceps.

CHEST PRESS. There are machines galore to do chest presses at every conceivable angle, but there is no need to get any fancier or more complicated than a barbell bench press, or even better, a dumbbell bench press. I say better because using dumbbells in this movement enables you to bring the weights lower than the plane of your chest, where you'd have to stop if using a barbell. A greater range of motion makes a more complete exercise. You'll have to use lighter weights than you could use doing them with a barbell as they are more difficult, but they are a better exercise. That being said, a barbell bench press is still a great pec, tricep, and front delt movement. As for incline and decline presses, they are great to do once in awhile. You should make the majority of your presses flat bench presses, but starting with your third chest workout do inclines, then do two more chest workouts with flat benches, then do declines.

Do not fall into the trap I see many people, mostly young men, fall into. They discover they can do more weight in a decline press, so they do mostly, or even exclusively, this type of chest press. And it is true that you generally can do more in a decline because this takes an inch or so off your range of motion and puts you in a more powerful position. In a year they look like they need a brassiere because their lower pecs are overdeveloped. Every fourth or fifth chest workout is adequate for declines.

FLYES. These are a better pure pec movement than even chest presses, as they do not directly involve the triceps. Again there are some great machines to perform these upon, and of these I very much prefer and recommend the prone machines over any seated variation, but they are probably best done with dumbbells, though a close second has to be cable flyes done on a cable crossover machine and a prone bench. Whatever type you do be absolutely certain to stretch the shoulders out thoroughly beforehand, and start conservatively as regards both amount of weight used and range of motion. At the bare minimum, wrists should cross at the top (for machine and cable flyes) or weights touch gently at the top (for dumbbell flyes) and should be lowered until either the weights or handles or pads are in a straight plane even with your chest. If you are limber enough to go lower, by all means try, but be careful. Lowering too much weight too far too fast is a classic way to tear your shoulder muscle or rotator cuff. If you do this it will plague you for years. Maybe forever.

OVERHEAD PRESS. Also commonly called a military press. They are one of the most basic and popular movements in all of weight training. They consist of simply moving a weight, be it a barbell, dumbbells or on a machine, from the shoulders straight up into the air nearly to lockout of the elbow joint, then back down to the shoulders again. If using a barbell do not lower the weight behind the neck – this can cause the very painful impingement syndrome just like pulldowns behind the neck can. Why run the chance of injury to yourself?. Lowering the weight behind the neck confers no advantage.

This is a particularly difficult lift for women. I have seen ladies, undeniably strong in all other lifts, unable to do an overhead press with anything but what would be considered a light weight. It is something structural no doubt, probably having to do with the size of the shoulders.

And it is actually the most difficult way to lift a weight - straight up, directly against gravity, with no or very little arc and no swing or momentum to assist. Though it is a strong tricep movement, I include it in workouts as the primary movement for the medial head of the deltoid (side of the shoulder). You've seen men and women with that strikingly attractive, very round, powerful look to the side of their shoulders. I guarantee they do these.

LATERAL RAISE. Also called 'lat' raises but not to be confused with lat pulldowns. Pulldowns are for your lats, more properly known as the latisimus dorsi muscles. The lat raise is another move for the medial deltoids, and so named because the weight is lifted laterally out away from the body. Though not the preeminent mass and strength builder that the overhead press is, it should be included in this workout, as it emphasizes the lower part of the range of motion of the medial delts. There are several good lat raise machines but there is no need to use anything more complicated than a set of dumbbells.

The starting and ending position is with the dumbbells held in front of the thighs with a *slight* bend in the elbows. This takes the stress off the joint. Raise them laterally out to your sides until your arms are parallel to the ground, keeping that same slight bend in the elbows. Viewed head-on your arms and shoulders should form a straight line. Do not throw your forearms up in the air like you are surrendering. Be sure to keep the thumb side of the weight angled down slightly. Think of pouring a pitcher of water with a greatly exaggerated motion. Lower and repeat. These start out easy enough but get hard very quickly, so begin with a conservative weight.

Though not directly involving chest or tricep muscles, they go hand in hand with the overhead press which does involve the tricep, so do them as part of this workout.

OVERHEAD TRI EXTENSION. To fully exercise the belly of the tricep you must do some form of overhead extension. These can be done standing but it's better to sit. Cup one head of a dumbbell with both hands and start with it held straight overhead to the fullest extension of your arms. Lower it as far as possible behind your head, then raise and repeat. Keep your elbows in close to the sides of your head! If you allow them to bow outwards you will crack yourself on the back of the head with the weight. However if you do them properly they are perfectly safe.

For some reason many people believe that this movement is redundant – a repetition of the overhead press. It is not. The difference is that in an overhead press you drive the weight straight up and your elbows travel in a shallow arc to the outside (his is what makes it such a good movement for the medial head of the delts), while in the overhead extension the arms from the shoulder to the elbows are stationary while the forearms act as levers to raise and lower the weight behind your head.

There are excellent machines for this movement, but they are rare. If you are fortunate enough to have access to one, <u>use it</u>. It is an exceptionally difficult machine but well worth learning to master. I worked one <u>hard</u> for a year and added nearly an inch to my arms with it. I now do the whole stack of three hundred pounds for reps. I am not a spokesman for any particular make of machine or workout gear and so won't give the brand-name of the machine I am speaking of here, but will happily endorse it verbally if asked.

PUSHDOWNS. Not to be confused with pressdowns, which basically emulate parallel bar dips while seated at a machine. They are performed at an overhead pulley station and can be done properly with nearly any handle, but a rope handle is the best. The exercise starts once you have brought the handle down from overhead and hold it in front of your collarbone with your elbows locked into your sides. It helps to hold yourself bent forward from the waist slightly and with slightly bent knees. Press the handle down in a straight line, with no arc, until your arms are fully extended and straight down. If doing it with a rope handle (highly recommended and more difficult) spread your hands apart slowly and evenly during this entire downward portion of the movement. Let it raise slowly and under control. If using the rope, let your hands come back together during this upward portion of the movement. Repeat.

Depending on your body geometry and positioning you may need to turn your head to one side to avoid hitting yourself in the face with the cable. I once walked around for an hour after doing these with a long black line on my face from grease on the cable, much to the amusement of my coworkers and gym members, who thought it funny to not tell me. Why was it that I loved working there?

KICKBACKS. These are another particularly good

tricep movement. They look easy but aren't. In fact, they are exceptionally difficult if done properly. For this reason, at least in the beginning, do them in combination with <u>one</u> of the previously mentioned tricep movements, not both.

Kneel on a flat bench with your weight supported on one knee and the opposite hand. Hook the toes of that leg over the end of the bench. The other foot should be flat on the floor. With your free hand pull a dumbbell up until the forward head is approximately in your armpit. Your elbow should be above your back and must stay there throughout this movement. Try not to twist your torso during the execution of these. Raise the weight back in an arc, keeping your upper arm immobile, until your arm is completely straight. Lower and repeat. Do not swing the weight at the bottom of this motion. If done strictly these can result in a ferocious pump in your arms, especially in combination with one of the other two tricep movements.

OTHER SPLITS

There are certainly other ways of dividing up your workouts, but I do believe the triple split outlined above is the best for one reason, efficiency. I often see many people doing other types of split routines, for example an upper body, lower body double split routine, or a chest/back, arms/legs double split routine. Lets examine the first of these.

The Upper/Lower Split Routine. This is probably the most common yet one of the least efficient types of split. With this routine the entire upper body is done in one workout. Lets see, this means a movement for pecs, preferably two, an isolation movement for triceps, preferably two, a movement for the medial head of the deltoids, preferably two, a movement for lats, preferably two, a movement for lower back, a movement for traps, a movement for the middle back muscles, a movement for biceps, preferably two, a movement for forearms, preferably two, a movement for abs, preferably two.

This is a minimum of ten movements and perhaps as

many as seventeen. If you take only *three* seconds per rep, allowing for a minute rest between sets, and based on three sets of ten, with two minutes between lifts, and it will usually be more than that on the average, as you drink water, use the restroom, set up the machine or put the weights on a bar, talk to your friends, or wait for the particular piece of apparatus you want to use to become free, this means a bare minimum of fifty-five minutes spent just in the weight training portion of this workout, if you move like a machine from lift to lift doing the 'minimal' workout wherein you perform 'only' ten movements. I hope that you will take at least ten minutes to warm up and stretch before embarking automaton-like on this workout. This makes this 'abbreviated' workout one hour and five minutes long. If you elect to do the much more complete version of this workout, with seventeen separate movements, you are then looking at ninety-one point five minutes of moving like clockwork from lift to lift, except that again you should be taking at least the additional ten minutes to warm up and stretch. That makes this workout one hour forty-one point five minutes long.

There is bad news and there is good news at this point. The bad news is that you still have to do the lower body portion of this double split. The good news is that if you do an abbreviated version of this part of the split it will be much shorter (how could it NOT be?). It would entail one heavy pressing movement for quads, one curling movement for hamstrings, one calf movement, preferably two. Why, this sounds very much like the Monday workout of the triple split, and it is, minus abs, and it will take you – if we use the same formula we used to figure the length of the upper body portion – twelve and a third minutes. Maybe you now begin to get a tiny sense of inequity in the lengths of your workouts on this type of split.

Even if we don't do an abbreviated lower body workout, but include thigh abductors and adductors, that adds only six minutes to this workout, for a total of eighteen point five minutes. Still very unequal. What this upper/lower split does is to combine the back/biceps portion with the chest/

triceps portion of the triple split method into one very long workout.

I've had clients that wanted to train on an upper/lower split like this, and do it in two half- hour sessions a week. Ain't happenin'. If your trainer does train you like this then they are shortchanging you on several very important lifts.

Chest/Back, Arms/Legs Double Split. In some ways this makes more sense than the Upper/Lower Double Split, but in other ways less. I am not going to analyze/formulate the time taken by the workouts in this method, because the main problem here manifests itself not by the clock, but in a different fashion. Consider:

The chest portion of the first part of this workout will entail at least some form of chest press, probably two or even three if you do inclines **and** declines (all involve triceps – an arm muscle) and some form of flye. The back portion will involve a compound rowing movement (involving the biceps – an arm muscle), a pulldown (involving biceps – an arm muscle), and then a low back movement, like the Roman Chair, shrugs (which will work the forearms if you do them right – and by this I mean **heavy**), maybe some form of pullover, and maybe on this particular workout a movement not covered in the triple-split – a rear delt flye.

On to the arms/legs division. An arm workout will entail forms of triceps isolation movements but remember you have already cooked your triceps anywhere from medium to well-done in the chest portion of your previous workout. An arm workout will also entail forms of biceps isolation movements. You have already worked your biceps, at least somewhat, in the back portion of your previous workout. To be a complete arm workout you must then do some forearm work. But here again, you should have already worked them fairly well, though perhaps incompletely, with shrugs, also part of the back portion of your previous workout. If I am sounding redundant here then I am getting my exact point across. This split causes duplication of lots of effort, on separate days. Yes, there is a little redundancy in the triple-split as I outlined it as well, but it is *within* the same workout and therefor does not impinge on the recovery period of an individual muscle or muscle group.

The leg portion of this division would simply be the leg workout of the triple-split (gee, we keep coming back to this), including abs since they don't fit well in the chest/back division.

But lets be real. Just because the triple-split is the most time efficient and least redundant of the splits that I have used, seen used, or have read about, does not mean that you should never diverge from it. If you plateau or just plain get *bored* with your routine you should do something different. For example I occasionally do a workout of nothing but biceps and triceps isolation movements. This has been beneficial and because I usually do it as my last workout before a break in training it does not have to throw your triple-split out of order.

And a break in training is not always a bad thing. A vacation from the gym wherein I do no weight lifting at all is essential to my outlook and attitude once in a great while. It also allows complete muscle recovery and sets me up for new gains when I return and hit the weights hard. But the benefits of a break in training are quickly outweighed by the negative aspects (i.e. muscle atrophy and strength loss) if the break is much more than a week in length.

TRAINING CYCLES

This is the shortest chapter yet the concept it contains is the very heart of this training method. The other two aspects, training frequency and training divisions are certainly important, but I say this is the most important part because just by taking this concept and applying it to any other routine, you will have created a progressive method, albeit a less efficient one, for gaining strength and muscle mass. It is elegant in it's simplicity, effective in it's application, and adaptable for every age and level of fitness.

All the lifts performed, with a couple of exceptions, are based on three sets of ten repetitions each. The exceptions are the movements for calves and abs. Forearms also, if you do specific lifts for this oft-times neglected muscle group. These muscles are also flexed and worked so often just in our day to day activities that they can be relatively inured to exercise. Consequently they need to be worked a bit harder with more reps, so we base the movements for these muscle groups on three sets of fifteen repetitions each.

This three sets of ten 'rule' tells us what weight we should be using in any lift. By the end of your third set of ten it should be very difficult to finish. If you fail, reaching temporary total muscle fatigue, on your final rep of your final set, that is ideal. If you fail halfway through your second set, you have selected a weight that is too heavy. If you can easily finish your three sets of ten then it is too light. Remember, you do not get stronger by lifting weights that are easy to lift. You get stronger by lifting weights that are hard to lift.

Now is the time for an important aside. Remember the stopwatch? I told you we'd get back to it. It is used to time your rest periods between sets. This is important.

I use one minute as standard for rest periods between sets for beginners and this works well for most of them. If you are someone that already has good muscle endurance and feel that this is too long for you, then try forty-five seconds. I know some good trainers that hold their people to rests of only thirty seconds, but I believe that this is too short a rest when you lift heavy and are pushing yourself hard like you will with this method of training.

Whatever period works for you, you **must** keep it consistent, hence the stopwatch. This is why: if you can lift, say, a hundred pounds for example, for three sets of ten, in any lift, but are not timing your rest periods, and next week you can do one hundred ten in the same lift, you have no idea if it is because you grew stronger or because you rested longer between sets. If you time your rest periods, always keeping them the same and can do more in any lift, you **know** it is because you have grown stronger.

When it becomes less challenging to finish three sets of ten while using good form and always keeping your rest periods the same length, then move up to three sets of twelve **with the same weight**. This should make it challenging again, sometimes for only a workout or two, but often for more.

When finishing three sets of twelve no longer challenges you, it is <u>only then</u> that you increase the weight. The increase should be modest, no more than five pounds for an upper body movement, and no more than ten pounds for a leg movement, and if it is possible with whatever apparatus you are using to make an increase of even less, it is a good idea to do less. While an increase in your bench press of only two pounds a week seems ridiculously small to most people, in one year you will add one hundred and four pounds to this lift, theoretically. That is not bad. And you will have done it safely, without tissue injury setting back your training by weeks or even months. I add the caveat 'theoretically' because you will undoubtedly 'plateau' during this year, perhaps more than once. How to deal with this is covered in a following section.

With this increase comes a reduction in the number of repetitions. We do not drop back to three sets of ten, but rather to three sets of eight.

Invariably my clients feel this heavier but shorter workout is easier than the previous one of three sets of twelve. It <u>is</u> easier even though the weight lifted per rep is greater, because the total volume of training has dropped, as illustrated in the following table.

First Cycle
Leg Press. Step One.

200 lbs. X 10 repetitions = 2000 lbs.
X 3 sets = 6000 lbs. total volume this lift.

Leg Press. Step Two.

200 lbs. X 12 repetitions = 2400 lbs.
X 3 sets = 7200 lbs. total volume this lift.

Second Cycle.
Leg Press. Step One.

210 lbs. X 8 repetitions = 1680 lbs.
X 3 sets = 5040 lbs. total volume this lift.

Leg Press. Step Two.

210 lbs. X 10 repetitions = 2100 lbs.
X 3 sets = 6300 lbs. total volume this lift.

Leg Press. Step Three.

210 lbs. X 12 repetitions = 2520 lbs.
X 3 sets = 7560 lbs. total volume this lift.

Note that the very first cycle has only two steps. This is because we always begin with the sets of ten - the gauge of how much weight we should be starting with in any lift. After this it is simply steps one, two, and three in every cycle.

We progressed from a total training volume of six thousand pounds to seven thousand five hundred sixty pounds. An increase in total training volume of one thousand five hundred sixty pounds for one lift is significant, and in just five simple steps. For an upper body lift the increase should not be more than about five pounds, and usually less than that, if possible, although once in awhile I have increased it by more when I was having a particularly strong day. As with anything, do what works, but be **safe.**

And yes, a two hundred pound leg press will be too light for many, but I use this figure merely to illustrate this concept. Besides, its far better to err on the side of caution, particularly in the beginning when you are still discovering your capabilities. Remember, it is always the three sets of ten rule that determines your actual starting weight.

I must emphasize here that there is no timetable involved with this progression. The increases must occur only when you no longer feel challenged to finish the three sets at that particular weight or that particular number of reps. However, in the very beginning it would not be unrealistic to progress at the rate of one step per week, but this rate of improvement will not continue for long. You can go back and read about enervation on pages nine through eleven for an explanation of why this happens. If you can continue to move up rapidly with this method then you did not use a heavy enough starting weight. Remember, you should barely be able to finish your final rep at any step of this cycle.

Notice that when cycling from twelve repetitions to eight you remove what is essentially a whole set of twelve reps from your workout, going from a total of thirty-six reps to a total of twenty-four. The focus then becomes bringing the total volume up by raising the number of reps back up to ten per set, then twelve. Then when this is no longer a challenge to finish you once again increase the weight and decrease the number of reps to eight. Again, there is no timetable associated with this. The increases occur only when you are ready to perform at a higher level and know you can handle an increase.

The cycles for calves and abs are exactly the same except based on three sets of fifteen reps, then upped to three sets of seventeen, then increasing the weight and dropping to three sets of thirteen, or if you're superstitious, twelve.

This is the number of reps and the pattern recommended for building strength, but again one of the true beauties of the cycled method is that it is infinitely adaptable. If you work out with the aim of increasing your muscular endurance rather than functional strength or power, then simply follow this same pattern based on a higher number of reps. All other rules apply. For instance, if you are doing a high rep workout based on three sets of twenty repetitions, you still need to be using a weight that will be a challenge to finish your last rep of your last set with. The weight you can finish a total of seventy-two reps with will be less than what you can complete a total of thirty-six reps with, I promise you. Your training cycle would then be something like twenty reps, then up to twenty-four, then increase the weight a few pounds and drop the reps down to sixteen. That is, a twenty – twenty-four – sixteen endurance cycle rather than the ten – twelve – eight power cycle for gaining strength.

Once in awhile you will experience workouts in which you will not be able to finish a set at the new greater weight or higher number of repetitions. At this point you have two options. You may either 'recycle' that particular lift, dropping back one or even two steps and begin again to bring your training volume back up, or you can recycle that entire workout. The later has the advantage of keeping your written training record simple, but will have you performing at less than optimal level in other lifts until the lagging muscle or muscle group is up to par. The former will keep the workout itself running more efficiently at the expense of complicating your record keeping, because you would then need to keep track of one lift in which you are doing sets of eight while all the other lifts in that workout are at sets of ten or twelve. You decide.

Methodical, adaptable, cyclical, progressive, easy to implement, easy to remember, and it works.

THE NEXT LEVEL

The movements covered in the Training Divisions section are great basic lifts, but there are alternates to nearly all of them. For example, alternates to dumbbell flyes performed lying on a flat bench would be standing flyes performed on a cable crossover, or of course one of the many types of good flye machines. Alternates to lat pulldowns are wide-grip chins, or as discussed before, machine pullovers, or dumbbell pullovers. Leg press alternatives are weighted lunges, hack squats, sissy squats, Smith machine squats, squats in the lunge position, or of course, squats.

My favorite alternate to the overhead press is handstand pushups. This is an unconventional and exceptionally difficult movement, but it is a real attention getter. People have asked me to train them after just watching me do these. **Never** attempt these initially without a spotter. If you can't lift the equivalent of your bodyweight in an overhead press for reps do not attempt them. Obviously, if you can't do a handstand don't attempt them at all.

The only lift that I can think of that there is really no safe and practical alternative to is the seated calf raise done on a machine. Theoretically one could place a barbell across the knees while seated and perform something similar, but notice I said *safe* alternative. This would not only be uncomfortable, it would be downright hazardous to your knees and legs, as it would cause severe bruising and perhaps actual tissue and/or joint damage to your knees with the weights you will work your way up to using the cycled training method.

To carry your cycled training to the next level you must develop alternates to all your lifts. If, because of unavailability of equipment, physical limitations, or whatever reason, you cannot perform alternates to every single thing, don't loose sleep over it. Keeping a couple of the same movements won't really hurt anything, though it won't help either. Do the best you can to develop alternates, because once you have become conditioned to your triple-split routine, you develop a second triple-split routine and alternate between them. For example:

Week One: Monday – Legs & Abs workout #1
             Wednesday – Back & Biceps workout #1
             Friday – Chest & Triceps workout #1

Week Two: Monday – Legs & Abs workout #2
             Wednesday – Back & Biceps workout #2
             Friday – Chest & Triceps workout #2

Week Three: Monday – Legs & Abs workout #1
             Wednesday – Back & Biceps workout #1
             Friday – Chest & Triceps workout # 1

     Cycling between two sub-routines for each workout will greatly delay the inevitable 'plateau'. This is when your progress curve levels out and becomes flat, or nearly so.

     Some clients have been with me long enough so that we have developed a **third** triple-split routine and alternate between the three of them. It takes <u>four weeks</u> to return to your original triple-split routine with this program. This works fine for those who are more advanced, but its too much for anyone that hasn't trained on the single and then the dual triple-split program for some time. Your workout schedule then looks like this:

Week One: Monday – Legs & Abs workout #1
             Wednesday – Back & Biceps workout #1
             Friday – Chest & Triceps workout #1

Week Two: Monday – Legs & Abs workout #2
             Wednesday – Back & Biceps workout #2
             Friday – Chest & Triceps workout #2

Week Three: Monday – Legs & Abs workout #3
                     Wednesday – Back & Biceps workout #3
                     Friday – Chest & Triceps workout #3

Week Four: Monday – Legs & Abs workout #1
                     Wednesday – Back & Biceps workout #1
                     Friday – Chest & Triceps workout #1

There is no point in getting more complex than this 'triple triple-split'. You are literally cycling your cycles at this point. Cycles within cycles within cycles. I didn't rack my brain to name this training method.

Eventually, even on a 'triple triple-split' training cycle, you will plateau because, as well as this does work, there is no training method or technique with which you will not plateau sooner or later. A training plateau is an inevitable point you will reach when improvement seems to not occur, and they can last for quite some time if you do not know how to deal with them. Many, many people stay on what is essentially a self-imposed training plateau because they are unwilling to change their workout routine. Others become discouraged and may quit working out altogether. Don't let this be you. When you do plateau it is then time to shock your muscles back into growth mode using one or more of the following 'jump-start' techniques.

WHEN YOU PLATEAU
(and you will)

There are several good techniques to use when you reach a point where your gains slow or seemingly quit coming altogether. Some of these are very basic, some are more complex. I make the distinction that a technique requiring the assistance of a training partner or partners is a complex technique. Whatever helps get you started making gains again, provided safety is maintained, is good. Do what works.

Plateaus are commonly experienced as a result of overtraining. It sounds counter-intuitive but as I mentioned before, a short break from training of say, not more than a week, will often be what is required to set you up for making new gains. We are kind to ourselves and refer to these little vacations as the 'consolidation phase'.

The most elementary and often most effective training technique to break through a plateau is to alter the order in which you do your workout. This may temporarily fly in the face of the heaviest-lift-first rule. So be it. Another very simple thing is to cut your rest periods. Trim fifteen or more seconds from them. But again, for purposes of strength building, there is no point or profit in making them less than thirty seconds long.

Also on the simple list: adding a fourth set to your routine. This is the only time I would recommend this, and when you are again making noticeable gains, revert to three sets. This can work and is not a big or complex change to regular cycled training.

Burns are a technique I love to use, though they are a temporary violation of your set number of reps. At the end of your last set reset the weight for something like forty percent less, then rep out to failure as quick as you can. It will burn.

The up fast, down slow method, a great jump-start technique, is a good way to lift all the time, and can be used with cycled training without violating any of its principles. You raise the weight like a powerlifter, quickly, with explosive power, activating your fast twitch muscle fibers. You then lower it, taking at least four times the number of seconds (basically the slower the better) it took to lift, thus using slow twitch muscle fibers. Dr. Fred Hatfield writes at length of this method and its efficacy in his excellent text, "Bodybuilding, A Scientific Approach". I strongly recommend this book, and actually anything Fred writes on strength training.

Compound sets are an effective technique. Though not exactly an elementary technique they don't fall into the 'complex' category. They combine a set of two different lifts performed back to back and counted as one set. Probably the most common compound set is to do a set of leg presses then immediately do a set of calf raises, probably on the same machine, then rest. This is one (compound) set. Repeat three times for your three sets. They can combine any two lifts though, not just ones for the same muscle group or bodypart. If three or more different lifts are combined into one set it is called a superset. More than four lifts in one set becomes a small circuit, which brings us to the next technique.

Circuit training. Do one set of each of your lifts without resting in between to complete one circuit. Do three circuits for your workout. Variations on this are:

A) Include interval training – in which you do not use your max weight or even count your reps. Instead you focus on continuing to perform reps for a set interval, say ninety seconds, for each of your lifts until the circuit is complete. In this method one circuit is usually enough.

B) Do the circuit as in A above but in between stations, or perhaps in between every two or three, hop on a stationary bike and pedal at high speed for one interval period.

C) Time yourself through one repetition of the complete circuit and the next time you attempt to better your time. This can be done for one, two, or three complete circuits.

D) Do not perform a specific number of reps instead continue to rep out to the point of total temporary muscle failure, then proceed to the next lift. This is grueling and needless to say, one circuit of this is enough also.

The super slow technique is an interesting one. I will go so far as to say that for many, it may be the most effective of the 'simple' jump-start techniques. I have witnessed a few very focused and disciplined individuals get very good results from it. Basically, you do only one set of ten reps of any lift but spend twenty seconds performing each rep, ten seconds up and ten seconds down. This is extremely demanding and difficult to do, and it activates a huge number of muscle fibers. You must, of course, select a weight that is less than what you would normally lift. How much less is determined simply by what you can barely finish the set with, a one set modification of the 'three sets of ten rule'. The major drawback to this and the main reason people tend to not stick with it for long is that you must be constantly counting to regulate your ten seconds up and ten seconds down, which is monotonous, and the slow pace can cause people to become bored with it. Mostly though, because they are hard. Although it is a totally viable and valuable workout method to use daily and indefinitely, for these reasons I find it most practical and useful as a plateau- breaking technique.

Cheating. I hesitate to include this, but it is actually an acceptable technique if done in the appropriate manner and at the right time. When you begin to fail at the end of your set, which is what will happen if you're using the correct weight, you simply use a little body English to impart momentum to the weight so that you can go beyond failure, then and only then. Use only enough extra motion to get the job done. Cheating in the wrong way is terribly common, and most often done unconsciously. There are people that cheat every rep of every lift they do. They may do this because they are ignorant of proper form, but usually its because they're lifting to build their egos instead of their muscles and they can move greater poundages this way. These are usually the same people that show no improvement in their physiques, even after sometimes years in the gym. They might as well stay home and play tiddlywinks for all the actual deep muscle stimulation they get. More importantly, they are courting injury.

Drop sets, also called stripped sets, are more efficiently done with a partner, though this is not absolutely essential, particularly if done on a machine with a weight stack, so I classify them as a 'marginally complex' technique. Perform your first two sets as normal but on your last set continue on until you cannot complete another rep, then drop or strip a little weight off the apparatus – not much, ten pounds maximum – and bang out a few more reps until you start to fail again. Strip off more weight, continue, repeat, etc, until you either can barely move, or there is no more weight to strip off the machine/bar.

Of course what usually happens at this time is that someone, probably attractive and of the opposite sex, will walk by, ignorant of the possibly thousands of pounds of total weight you have just lifted, and watch pityingly as you, gasping with effort and with muscles bulging, struggle mightily to complete a rep with ten pounds.

Drop sets are very closely related to the next technique.

Forced reps fall into the 'complex' category as they require the assistance of a training partner or spotter. Perform your first two sets as normal but on your last set rep out until you begin to fail. At this point your spotter gives you manual assistance, just enough to complete several more reps, however many you need to reach total muscle failure. These are closely related to the next technique.

Negatives are a useful and productive 'complex' technique. You begin with a weight that is something on the order of forty to fifty percent more than you can lift alone. Your spotter helps you to lift the weight every rep but you lower it by yourself. Negatives can give dramatic results but are too demanding to perform regularly. The large weights handled are taxing to both the skeletal muscles and the joints and so they should be performed no more than necessary to shock your muscles back onto a growth curve. They also have a distinct tendency to cause muscle soreness. All of these considerations for negatives hold true but times two or three for the next technique.

Static training, another 'complex' technique, is somewhat akin to negative training but is more similar to isometrics, with one huge difference. In isometrics the weight is held motionless in the weakest part of the repetition while in static training it is held motionless in the portion of the lift in which you are strongest, shy of lockout. Enormous weights can be handled in this manner. Your spotter(s) bring the weight up to a predetermined point, usually just shy of lockout, and you then hold it motionless for a set, strict period of time, usually only up to a maximum of fifteen seconds. This is another time where a stopwatch becomes essential. When the weight moves down, even a quarter inch, the lift (actually a hold) is done. When it can be held for the full interval, it is time to up the weight, by a conservative amount. There are some important considerations when doing these:

A) Two spotters are sometimes required for this method. Due to the extremely heavy weights used, one man to spot for you, even a very large, strong man, is often not enough. For example, the guy who popularized static contraction training claims a static hold in the leg press of sixteen hundred pounds, and I do not believe this is an impossible weight for a strong man with this method.

B) Again, due to the extremely heavy weights used, your selection of equipment is crucial. For example, perform a static bench press or a squat with a Smith machine or in a squat cage, with the safety bars set appropriately, rather than with totally free weights. Other than when you first lift it into position, there is no range of motion in a static hold, so the slight superiority conferred by free weights for building power simply does not exist with this type of training, and the safety factor inherent in most machines is a major consideration. The main problem that then arises is that the type of machines that have a weight stack (as opposed to   machines on which you have to actually manually load weight plates) do not have enough weight on them for a strong person to be challenged with in a static hold, at least in some lifts. You must be innovative then, but not at the expense of safety.

C) Some other lifters, trainers, authors, etc. advocate this method as a total alternative to a more standard work out (i.e. cycled training). I have trained myself and others with static holds and believe that it is most valuable as I present it here, as a 'jump-start' method of working through a sticking point in your training.

Just remember that these techniques work best when used infrequently. They can and will shock your muscles back into growth mode, but you can't continue to shock them for very long.   These are overload techniques and are very hard on your body if used too often. At best, overuse of them quickly leads to overtraining. This has the effect opposite of that desired when your progress comes to a screeching halt as your body tries to rest and protect itself from the trauma. At worst, overuse of them will lead to injury.

Approach these with the attitude that they are for special and occasional use only, when faced with the dreaded plateau, and observe all safety considerations. Above all, use your head. Gyms really are one place where common sense rules.

NUTRITION

This is a training manual, not a diet book or food guide, but nutrition plays such a critical part in gaining strength, muscle mass, and general health and fitness, that it would be remiss to not include a section on it.

There are micronutrients – nutrients needed in very small amounts, and there are macronutrients – nutrients needed in comparatively large amounts.

Micronutrients are all the individual vitamins, minerals, enzymes, cultures, and trace elements. There are a lot of these and it is beyond the scope of this simple training manual to try to address each of them, but I'll address some important points.

Macronutrients are water, carbohydrates, protein, and fats. I also like to include dietary fibers, though technically they are just indigestible forms of carbohydrate.

On vitamins and minerals: Taking a daily multivitamin/multimineral tablet is cheap insurance against a deficiency. Note that I said multivitamin/multimineral, not simply multivitamin. Unless you have the necessary minerals in your system, your body will not be able to make use of the vitamins.

I hear from so many people "Well I prefer to get my vitamins from the food I eat," and I heartily agree with that sentiment, but do you know anyone who eats a perfect balance of perfect food every day? I don't. But do remember that supplements are exactly that, supplements, meant to supplement the food in your diet. They are not food themselves, and do little or no good if taken on an empty stomach.

Some of the better multis also contain many of the other micronutrients and even herbs. Read the labels and get the most complete one you can find.

As important as vitamins and minerals are, enzymes may be as important. The best way to insure you're getting adequate enzymes is through the consumption of raw, fresh, fruits and vegetables. Cooking, heating, canning, and processing destroys them.

Live beneficial bacteria cultures are present in yogurt and kefir and are a boon to intestinal health. I recommend the daily consumption of yogurt, especially after eating meat. It helps retard spoilage in your digestive system. Yes, you read that correctly. Meat can spoil inside your stomach.

Meat, particularly red meat, is one of the slower and more difficult things for your body to digest, usually taking at least a couple days to pass through your system. If you eat a large amount of it at once some will remain undigested long enough for it to begin to putrefy before it is assimilated and/or eliminated. I found this difficult to believe, like you probably, but consider the following common sense argument.

What would happen if you thoroughly chewed up a big steak, mixing the mouthfuls of masticated meat with saliva, spit them into a waterproof bag, added some digestive juices to liquify it, then let it sit for a couple of days in heat equal to body temperature, ninety-eight point six degrees? Conjures up a pretty disgusting picture, eh? This is what can happen in your digestive tract. Anything that can help keep this internal spoilage from occurring is certainly something you should consider making a part of your diet.

Don't let this put you off meat. It is wonderful protein, contains other valuable nutrients, and is delicious. Just enjoy it in small to medium-sized portions, perhaps take a good digestive enzyme afterward, and end that meal with a couple big spoonfuls of yogurt.

On herbs. If you like them, take them - once you've educated yourself about them. Some herbs can have adverse effect and you don't want to just take them randomly. I've taken various herbs over the years for various reasons and had some good results with some of them, none with others. I continue to take a couple different herbs, and I keep a couple others on hand for occasional and specific use. Herbs have been used as medicine for thousands of years, by billions of people, and I don't believe they're all wrong. Strictly speaking though, there is no nutritional requirement for herbs and herbal supplements.

All the macronutrients are essential for life, but first and foremostly is water. So much has been written about adequate water intake that I don't need to go on at length about it, but it is so important that I will make a few points:

A) <u>Nothing</u> happens in the human body without water. That is, nothing except death by dehydration. Every other physical process in the body requires water.

B) It seems that the thirst response is rather weak in most people. Humans are rather poorly 'wired' in this respect. By the time a person actually feels thirsty they are already well on the way to being dehydrated. The simple, easy, and effective rule for drinking enough water is to drink water often enough so that you never feel thirsty.

C) A reduction of even a couple percent of your water weight can have serious detrimental effects on your health and performance. As far as your weight training, it can cause muscle weakness, cramps, and tremors, none of which you can afford in your quest for strength. Drink water upon waking because you have lost blood volume due to dehydration via respiration while you are asleep. Coffee, tea, soda, fruit juice, beer, protein drinks, etc. are not substitutes for water.

D) Bottled water is generally better water than tapwater, but not always. The word 'springwater' on the label of a bottle of water is no guarantee of purity. Basically all water, unless it is rainwater, glacier water, or desalinated seawater, comes from a spring somewhere. It could be piped in from the river bottom in the middle of the city, poured into a jug and rightfully be called springwater. 'Springwater bottled at the source' is at least a somewhat better indicator of water quality and purity.

E) For the reasons mentioned, some people will drink distilled water. This has its pros and cons. Distilled water is as pure as any water practically available unless you have access to water purified through reverse-osmosis process. Certainly pure water is a good thing, but it is important to take into consideration that because of this utter purity, distilled water lacks minerals that other waters normally contain and so will actually draw, or 'leach' water-soluble minerals from your body, much more so than the consumption of normally mineral-laden water.

Fats used to be thought of as the bogeyman of everyone that sought optimum health. A terribly underweight lady even once told me that I was killing myself with my lecithin supplements because "you know of course that lecithin is a type of fat." She made it sound like a dirty word. A kind of anti-fat mania swept the fitness and nutrition world and it lasted for quite awhile. Thank goodness this insanity is mostly behind us now. Yes, saturated fats and trans-fats should be avoided whenever possible, but there are nutritional fats that are absolutely required for good health. These are the omega three, six (in moderation), and nine fatty acids. Fats can also be an important energy source, but don't load up on them on the excuse that you need them to work out, because even the 'good' fats are extremely calorie dense.

Generally, the rule of thumb is that if a fat is solid at room temperature it is a saturated fat (i.e. lard, beef tallow, pork rind) and generally should be avoided. If it is liquid at room temperature (i.e. olive oil, flaxseed oil) usually it is unsaturated fat and you can and should have some, in moderation. There are exceptions to this so **read labels** when buying dietary oils. The healthy oils can actually have the effect of lowering your blood cholesterol level.

It was proven quite some time ago that the consumption of saturated fat causes a much greater increase in blood cholesterol level than the actual consumption of dietary cholesterol. In other words, it isn't the eggs you eat for breakfast that are the big problem. The butter or bacon grease they were fried in is the real culprit. Surprisingly, eggs are still demonized by many for their cholesterol content and I've had people admonish me for my consumption of this fine food.

Carbohydrates are the preferred fuel of the body. The best source of complex carbs is whole grain. Whole grains are a wonderful long-term energy source and also contain fiber and a small amount of protein. Simple carbs (sugars and starch) are 'empty' calories, in and of themselves having no other value as foods and you can live just fine forever without any at all. The easy rule of thumb to tell a complex from a simple carb is this: If its white its a simple carb. With the exception of dairy products, avoid white foods. Plain white rice, plain white pasta, plain white bread, plain white peeled potatoes, are essentially all simple carbs. Much healthier alternates to these extremely popular foods are brown or wild rice, whole wheat pasta or spinach pasta, dark whole grain breads, and potatoes with the skin. Carbs are usually inexpensive, have a long shelf life, are easy to store, easy to fix, easy to digest and generally taste pretty good, which is why so many people get more carbs than they need, and far too much starch and sugar in particular. In comparison, protein is more expensive, more difficult to prepare, and more difficult to digest, though it can taste wonderful, like a good filet mignon for example. To make it easy to get and assimilate enough protein, a good high quality protein powder, mixed into a convenient shake can be useful. The best are those that are a mix of casein and whey protein. This mix has high bioavailability, and is both a long and short term protein source for your body's maintenance and recovery. Whey alone digests and metabolizes very quickly and is not a good long term protein source. Almost as good and considerably less expensive are milk and egg protein powders. Soy protein is good protein for women but be aware you will have to combine this with the intake of whole grains to get the complete amino acid profile you need for it to be usable by your body. If you are a soy protein user take an l-lysine supplement as it lacks this essential amino acid. Soy also has some anti-carcinogenic effects that are beneficial, particularly for females, though this is not the only reason I recommend it only for them. Soy, be it protein powder, soy milk, or tofu, can have 'estrogenic' effects. *Feminizing* effects. Men - well, *most* men - will want to avoid this.

For a useful and interesting viewpoint on vegetarian bodybuilding the legendary Bill Pearl is a font of information.

He also has a training manual called simply "Getting Stronger" that is excellent. Bill is a rare specimen: a vegetarian who is also a champion bodybuilder and noted for being a very strong guy. He is also a native American, for some reason also a rarity in bodybuilding circles.

Protein is what you are made from, except for bones, teeth, and fat cells. For someone weight training three times a week as outlined in this manual, consuming a gram of protein a day per pound of lean bodyweight is good..

Your lean bodyweight is simply your weight minus the weight of your bodyfat. This is determined by a bodyfat measurement, which a good trainer can do for you. The fancy electronic hand-held devices that purport to measure bodyfat are notoriously inaccurate and in my opinion not worth the plastic they're made of. Even the very high-end bathroom scales with this feature are not worthy of consideration.

I was once approached by my friend George, a tall, broad, elderly man, healthy and in good shape. He was very troubled because his well-meaning son had given him an expensive, name-brand bathroom scale that also measured bodyfat electronically, and it showed that he had nearly forty percent bodyfat. He's a fine fellow but has perhaps a little too much blind faith in technology. I quickly had him in my office for a manual measurement and a reading of nineteen percent - not bad for a big man in his eighties - quickly calmed his fears. Situations just like this occur regularly.

For all but clinical/scientific purposes, these manual skinfold measurements give a reading that is quite accurate and can then be used to determine your lean bodyweight, and from that your daily protein requirements.

For example, if you weigh two hundred pounds and have ten percent bodyfat this equals twenty pounds of bodyfat. Subtracting this figure from your total bodyweight gives you the figure of one hundred eighty pounds. This is your lean bodyweight, and it is equal to the total number of grams of protein you need to consume daily to actually build some muscle at this level of training.

Many will protest this and say it is too much protein.

This is another time you must consider the source. In my experience those most adamant about this are usually either underweight people who don't eat enough to begin with, or overweight people who prefer their calories in the form of simple carbohydrates. If the human body were one hundred percent efficient at digesting and assimilating protein, you could eat far less and grow muscle, but it isn't. In fact, its not even close.

There are bodybuilders and powerlifters that consume up to two and a half times that much (or two and a half grams of protein per day per pound of lean muscle mass) to maintain and build their enormous physiques. I think this is overkill, but I'm not a three hundred pound man whose main goal in life is to squat a thousand pounds.

RANDOM MUSINGS OF A GYM RAT

Why I love being a trainer.

I love weight training and gyms and generally speaking the people that work out in them. Gyms, probably like any other establishment that deals with the public, are full of characters, personalities and egos, some of them quite colorful and humorous. By and large they all have one thing in common. They are interested, for one reason or another, in improving their health and fitness level. With some the focus is increasing their strength and power. Others are there to improve their athletic performance. Some strive to build and sculpt their bodies into an aesthetic ideal. Frequently people work out to overcome a serious health problem, or to rehab an injury. Many, many folks are there to loose weight.

My favorite people are the ones that come in wide-eyed and timid, never having been in a gym before in their lives, wanting to join, eager to improve themselves, but without a clue as to how to go about it.

It is appropriate to reiterate here that safety is **always** the first consideration. The single most important thing you can ever do for someone new is to show them the correct, safe way to work out.

These folks are fertile soil and only need the right seed planted in them to bloom. No instruction, or worse yet, wrong instruction can really screw them up, perhaps hopelessly. I always strive to treat these folks with respect, understanding, and a genuine interest in making sure their initial experience in my gym is a positive one. A bit of courtesy, consideration, and a sense of humor also go a long way, but more than anything you have to honestly care about these new people, your clients, and all the gym folks that come up to you for a bit of information or encouragement. As a trainer I have always refuted the saying that "practice makes perfect". This is very wrong! Practicing anything incorrectly only ingrains incorrect form in your mind. Only perfect practice makes perfect, and it is your responsibility to impart perfect technique and form, and thus safety and efficacy, to these people.

Something that always upsets me is when I see trainers and gym owners that regard clients as cattle, and training as strictly a numbers game. You've seen the ones I'm talking about. Their focus is to get the clients in, give them only as much time and attention as they pay for and not a bit more, then get them the heck out and hustle the next warm body in. Don't ever try to ask one of these trainers for advice about anything unless you're their client and it is during your appointment, because you'll usually get no more than a stony stare and a mumbled reply along the lines of ". . .uh, I don't have time to talk about it right now." Maybe you'll be ignored entirely or coldly told that their time isn't free. In many cases gym management is to blame for this, but in many cases trainers **are** part of gym management.

I don't know how these trainers keep clients because this is the worst P.R. imaginable. Sure, if they're energetic and visible they'll attract some clients initially, but they don't get the repeat customers they could with a little consideration. I am only as busy training people as I care to be, so perhaps my perspective on this is somewhat different than many trainers. My day in the gym begins at a very early hour when not as great a number of people want to train, but in spite of this, the largest percentage of my clients have stayed with me for a long period of time, some for several years.   They're extremely loyal to me, but only because I'm loyal to them and have a genuine concern for their welfare.

A trainer has such a golden opportunity to do so much more for a client besides just build their bodies, if they will just make the effort to get to know them a little. You can have such a positive effect on a clients attitude, perception, self-esteem, self-confidence, even their peace of mind. Clients honor me by asking for my thoughts and insight on everything from career changes and relationship issues to child rearing, not because I'm an authority on these things, but because they have come to regard me as a friend and they value my opinions and counsel. I am very proud and happy of the fact that, while my clients are incredibly important to me as clients, most of them are better friends to me than anything else. Its a <u>great</u> job if you're me!

A trainer definitely has to be a people person. If you're not you have no business being a trainer because, after all, it is the people business we are in, in a very pure sense. A trainer must be personable, caring, and interested in helping people. It is wonderful and gratifying that people put so much faith in me and entrust me with such an important part of their health. It is a privilege to be a trainer and I strive to always remember that and be the best one I can be.

And being a trainer is such a unique job! It is the one facet of health care that doesn't require a medical degree, and its also the only job I know of where the person paying you does all the work. They even thank you for making them exert themselves.

People, in all their wonderful variety, have always fascinated me, and the gym is a wonderful place to observe and meet them. I've already written of some interesting individuals in this book, and there are so many others that I can't begin to recount all of them to you, but I will make mention of one inspiring individual, my dear friend Joyce McDonald.

When I began working with her she was only able to curl a set of three pound dumbbells for three sets of ten reps, but within a year of cycled training was using a pair of twelve pounders. This is the example of a four hundred percent increase in functional strength that I mentioned earlier. She could also do lat pulldowns with eighty pounds. No, these weights will never go down in the annals of gym lore as anything spectacular, but when I tell you that she was only five feet tall and that she turned <u>ninety-three</u> during our sixth month of training, it puts it in the proper perspective. Age alone is no excuse for not exercising.

Other benefits of weight training.

Aside from the obvious positive physical effects of weight training, and exercise in general, there are other advantages that might not be readily apparent.

First and foremost of these more intangible benefits is stress relief. Vigorous physical activity is one of the very best ways to decompress. When the pressures of job, family, relationships, money, time, and life in general get to be a bit too much, it is time to concentrate on what you do have control over: your body and your workouts. Training hard demands focus and attention and if you give it one hundred percent then at least this time is time not spent worrying. Working out can be very freeing in this way. One can achieve an almost zen-like state of being while moving the heavy iron, a meditative mind-set, or more accurately, the lack of a mind-set. Those that meditate regularly understand what I mean by this. It is a break from earthly troubles and concerns and this hiatus helps with perspective and in restoring a measure of serenity and peace of mind.

Many times I have begun my workouts burdened by a mind full of woes, some trivial, some not so trivial, some imagined, some very real. Forty-five minutes later I exited the gym, sweating, exhausted, spent, and panting, yet strangely refreshed and calmed, with better focus and perception about what is really important.

Some say it is because of the endorphins that are released during intense exercise. Others claim that working out hard is like paying penance and redeems them, at least in their own eyes. I prefer to utilize instead of analyze, and just let it provide me whatever benefit it may. That it does provide a mental benefit I have no doubt whatsoever. Beyond that I feel it provides an emotional and even a spiritual benefit as well.

Strength training is a *value added* pastime, though of course for many it goes far beyond a mere pastime. It can actually become a way of life. It is recreation, stress relief, anti-aging therapy, and preventative medicine all in one. Compare this to both the long and short-term benefits of other common pastimes like video games, watching television, surfing the net, pub crawling, getting high, or reading tabloids. Value added? You decide.

There is strong, and then there is <u>STRONG</u>.

When it comes to strength and strong people I've seen some amazing things, both in and out of the gym, and know of several others. I love stories of old time and modern day strongmen and have accumulated a small library on the subject. Here are some of my personal favorites. I find these very inspirational and motivating. The facts as I present them are true to the best of my knowledge and research.

There was a Canadian years ago by the name of Arthur Dandurand who could pick up a V-8 engine, cradle it before him in his arms and walk fifty paces before slowly setting it down. There is an account of Dandurand's strength written by non other than Joe Weider, who knew him personally. As a youth Joe worked out in the same gym as Arthur. One day Dandurand asked him to pick a bar up off the floor and bring it to him, but the husky youth couldn't budge it. It was filled with lead. Arthur then proceeded to pick the bar up off the floor with one hand and carry it straight-armed across the gym and place it in a rack. Dandurand was a short, stocky man, a pocket-sized Hercules, much like Fred Hatfield, or Franco Columbu.

Contrary to the prevailing notion, tall people do **not** have a leverage advantage. In fact they are at a <u>disadvantage</u> when it comes to lifting heavy weight. This is not to say that a lanky person cannot be strong. They can, and I know several, but it is just more difficult for those with this type of body structure.

At six feet one and about one hundred seventy-five pounds, Dr. Ray Koury is certainly the polar opposite of stocky, but as I wrote before, I have seen him go 'ass to ankles' in the squat with five hundred pounds, for reps.

But the fact is that stocky men have a distinct advantage when it comes to raw power, due to their body structure. Short, thick arms and legs have a huge leverage advantage over long, slender ones.

One of the strongest men I personally know - and I know many - is Steven 'Bear' Dickerson, cousin to Mr. Olympia Chris Dickerson. He is of medium height and has extremely thick limbs and a fifty-eight inch chest. Once when I was in the process of moving I watched Bear pick my sofa up *by one end* and walk out to the moving van with it sticking straight out in front of him. A man of equal mass but taller and longer-limbed could not have done this. Power. Leverage. Not surprisingly, he excelled at both powerlifting and Olympic lifting.

To give you some idea of the amount of raw explosive power he possesses in his massive frame: I saw him shatter the mechanism at the carnival with which you ring the bell by hitting the teeterboard with a sledge. I've also seen him crack walnuts in the crook of his twenty-two inch arm, and break a bathroom scale by squeezing it. It is also always fun to take him to the 'guess your weight' booth at the fair. "Well, big fella you go about two-fifty," they tell him, then he proceeds to tilt their scales at well over three hundred pounds. I've never seen anyone guess within fifty pounds of Bear's true bodyweight. He does look like a big man, but doesn't appear anywhere near as massive as he actually is.

Muscle weighs more per unit of volume than fat and when a large percentage of your bodyweight is muscle you will weigh more than you look, and this is not a bad thing. For a practical example, if forced to defend yourself, God forbid, it is far better for a foe to greatly underestimate your mass and strength. This can be a huge hidden advantage. People usually think I weigh around one hundred eighty-five pounds. As of this writing I am two hundred twenty and occasionally go a few pounds more. This has availed me well and surprised sparring opponents during martial arts (Jeet Kune Do) instruction. Greater solid body mass means a greater ability to absorb the shock of blows. It also makes it more difficult for an opponent to knock you down.

I must emphasize one thing here however. Strength alone does not win fights and a little weight training can be a dangerous thing if it gives you a false sense of invulnerability and makes you cocky. Trust me, you don't want to piss off an experienced street fighter or seasoned martial artist with a display of muscle and machismo.

I strongly recommend a book entitled "Bouncers Guide to Barroom Brawling." by Peyton Quinn. Mr. Quinn is for real. He knows his business and this no b.s. guide can save many a brash youngster from a world of hurt; physical, legal, and otherwise.

Three time Mr. Olympia, Franco Columbu began weight training to gain strength for boxing, and gain strength he did. In fact he gained so much that he later nearly killed an opponent in the ring. He decided then and there to leave fighting and devote himself full time to bodybuilding and powerlifting. He is one of only a few pro bodybuilders who was also a successful powerlifter. He did an official seven hundred seventy pound deadlift in competition, at a bodyweight of less than two hundred pounds. He could pick up the front of a car, hang from a bar by his toes, and blow a hot water bottle up like a balloon. His training partner, Arnold Schwarzenegger, said he was convinced that for his size Franco was the strongest man in the world, and Arnold was himself no slouch when it came to moving the heavy iron. The Austrian Oak could cheat curl a two hundred fifty pound barbell and bench press over four hundred pounds.

"Dr. Squat", Fred Hatfield, at forty-five years old and weighing two hundred fifty-five pounds, squatted one thousand fourteen pounds, more than anyone ever in an official powerlifting competition at that time. The list of his accomplishments in the world of strength training is long and impressive. As mentioned before, his many fine books and articles contain excellent and precise explanation of how muscles work and how to make them grow, backed by scientific research, studies, facts, and figures, not anecdotes and opinions. I've come to know Fred a bit and am constantly impressed with his formidable intellect, vast knowledge of many diverse subjects, his deep faith, and his sincere dedication to his friends and loved ones. An example of a true Renaissance man.

Least anyone think I'm ignoring the fairer sex in these remembrances of amazing feats of strength, I think it is only fitting to mention that the world record for one arm chin-ups is held by a woman. Not one **handed** chin-ups – in which you grip the bar with one hand and hold onto the wrist of that hand with the other – but one arm doing all the work. Diminutive circus performer Lillian Leitzel cranked out **twenty-seven** back in 1918, a record that to my knowledge has never been surpassed by anyone of either sex. Think you're strong? Next time you're at a chin-up bar try to do one from a dead hang. Just do yourself a favor and try this when no one else is around.

Jill Mills is another amazingly strong lady, and another of those rather rare individuals who is a successful powerlifter and bodybuilder. She has squatted with six hundred twenty-two point seven pounds, a woman's world record in her weight class. She can also bench three hundred eighty-five pounds, and deadlifts five hundred fifty-one. I've spoken with Jill and attest that while she does indeed look strong, she is a feminine and pretty lady.

Ian 'Mac' Batchelor, an L.A. bartender, was the undisputed arm wrestling champion of the world for *twenty-five years*. He never lost a match. Ever. Name any pro athlete in any sport who ever had a record like that for a greater length of time. Yes, yes, Rocky Marciano was undefeated heavyweight boxing champ of the world, an incredible athlete and genuine tough guy, but his career didn't last a quarter of a century. In the realm of hand and grip strength Mac had no equal. He could put a bottlecap (an old-time steel bottlecap, not one of the little tin caps used in later years) between each finger of both outstretched hands and squeeze his fingers together laterally, bending the bottlecaps in half. He could also hold an iron manhole cover out palm down in a pinch grip between thumb and fingers of one hand. Mac *looked* like an old-time strongman, with an enormous three hundred pound frame and a big, dark, handlebar moustache that he kept waxed and curled up on the ends. Incidentally, Mac used squats extensively in his workouts. Hmm . . .

At seven feet nine inches tall and five hundred eighty pounds in weight, Angus MacAskill was the largest non-acromegalic giant known to have ever lived, and the stories of his incredible feats of strength seem to contradict what I wrote earlier about tall men being at a disadvantage in lifting great weight. The fact that he was not an acromegalic giant might account for some of this. This means that he did not have a pituitary disorder that caused him to be afflicted with clinical giantism. The unfortunate individuals that suffer from this condition have exaggerated features such as limbs or other bodyparts grown out of proportion with their torsos, prognathous jaws, supraorbital ridges, are physically weak, generally suffer from a host of other health disorders, and die an early death. Angus suffered none of these things. He was simply an <u>extremely</u> large guy, with good proportion and features. I've seen a photograph of him and this and other likenesses show that he was a broad-shouldered, powerfully-built man, but essentially normal-looking in all but size. I strongly suspect he was also one of those men blessed with superior enervation and tendon strength, as discussed earlier.

He once set a forty foot mast in place in a ship "as easily as a farmer sets a fence pole", but the most famous story of his great strength is that of him lifting a ship's anchor and walking down the pier with it on a bet, though there is question about what it actually weighed. Many say it weighed two thousand seven hundred pounds, but most ship anchors in the area at the time weighed less than this, si its likely this has been exaggerated in the telling over the years.

In Cape Breton, Nova Scotia where he lived, the streets were rivers of mud when it rained. One wet day a team of draft horses pulling a freight wagon bogged down and stuck fast in the road. For a dollar Angus pulled the whole rig out by himself. As a young man he was seen more than once casually strolling down the street with a three hundred pound barrel of pork under *each* arm.

A bare-knuckle boxing champ toured the area, offering a

substantial cash prize to anyone who could go a single round with him. Angus was by nature a peaceful man with no interest in fighting, but the man taunted him unmercifully, a very unwise thing to do. Angered, the giant finally entered the ring and when the champ took his hand for the customary pre-fight handshake Angus simply crushed his hand, ending his career. Witnesses said that blood shot from the man's fingertips when Angus squeezed it. Another time a drunken three hundred pound ship captain tried to goad him into a wrestling match and Angus refused, more than once. Finally Angus had enough of the bully's jeering. He grabbed the huge man and threw him over a woodpile ten feet high.

He was much more than a local character and strongman however. He bought property, opened a mill and general store, and became a respected merchant and gentleman, widely known for his business acumen and generosity. He disliked selling on credit but would not let a hungry person leave his store without food. The term 'pillar of the community' is an appropriate description of Angus – in many ways! There exists today in Nova Scotia the Giant MacAskill Museum where many artifacts and much information about this legendary strong man can be studied.

Though of a later era, Louis Cyr was still another incredible Canadian strongman and was one of those rare individuals blessed with strength from birth. He became known as the strongest man in Canada at seventeen when he bested the titleholder in a contest that consisted of lifting heavy boulders. The champion hefted a four hundred pound boulder, his best lift. Young Louis then shouldered one weighing nearly five hundred pounds to win decisively.

He once picked up a weight weighing a maximum of either five hundred fifty-three or five hundred eighty-eight pounds with *one finger*. I found both figures listed for the famous one-finger lift. Maybe he did both. For a time, part of his act was to hang a rope ladder from one finger over the edge of an elevated platform while his wife climbed up it. I've seen an old poster depicting them performing this feat and it showed the ladder hanging from his pinkie and at arm's length away from his body. Whether this is accurate and true I have no way of knowing, but with a man of his strength perhaps it is.

In his most famous show of strength he had *two* draft horses fastened to each arm. The conditions of this contest were simple: the horses could not be whipped into lunging forward, and Louis had to hold his clenched fists butted together in position across his chest with no grasping or interlocking of fingers. The animals were given a gentle giddyap but his arms remained immobile. They strained against their harnesses until they dislodged clods of earth with their hooves, but Louis remained as immobile as a statue, some said for several minutes. In another exhibition he pushed a railroad car on the tracks, *uphill*. He performed these and many other shows of great strength before scores of credible witnesses and some were recorded in photographs.

Louis, like many other very large, strong men, was an endo-mesomorph, with a large belly and an appetite to match. He was a world class trencherman, and his capacity for food was legendary. It is said that he ate more than four normal men. Unfortunately Cyr also had something of a temper. This, combined with his awesome physical power, made him a dangerous man at times. While still a young boy he once beat up a gang of fourteen ruffians who had antagonized him by making fun of his long flowing hair, of which he was inordinately proud.

While its certain that the giant MacAskill was also a super-strong human being, some of the stories of his life and feats of strength at times probably cross into the realm of legend. Cyr's accomplishments were so well witnessed and recorded that there is little doubt about any of them. He was certainly the strongest man of the nineteenth century whose feats were reliably documented.

Bruce Randall, whom I mentioned briefly before in the section on lower back training, was also a remarkable strong man. Bruce was a Marine and while stationed overseas he decided to take full advantage of the station mess hall and gym and devoted himself to weight training and eating. In something like a year and a half he took his bodyweight from one hundred ninety-eight pounds to four hundred one pounds and his strength, not inconsiderable to begin with, grew accordingly. At his peak of weight and power he was supposedly capable of a good morning with eight hundred pounds. In spite of having witnessed some phenomenal lifts of various sorts over the years I find this almost unbelievable. However, I do have a photo of him performing this movement with six hundred pounds, itself an incredible weight, so I will say that if an eight hundred pound good morning could've ever been performed by anyone, it was Bruce Randall at four hundred one pounds.

This is really more akin to an old-time strong man stunt and, despite this interesting historical aside, the efficacy of this movement as a lower back exercise is far outweighed by the inherent risk of severe neck and back injury. Let me make this very clear: I do NOT recommend doing good mornings. In fact I recommend **not** doing them.

Upon returning stateside Bruce left the military and in fairly short order slimmed down to two hundred twenty pounds and took first at the Mr. America contest that year. Photos taken at that time show a lean and defined physique. All this in the space of about two years.

I mentioned Paul Anderson earlier but a better telling of his accomplishments is required. In the annals of strength he has no equal. During his lifting career he broke or established almost every strength and lifting record that existed.

At the 1955 World Championships in Moscow he competed against the holder of the overhead press world record, the Russian lifter Medvediev. Medvediev, looking like a bodybuilder with a narrow waist, barrel chest, and low bodyfat, went first. He struggled but succeeded in equaling his record lift of three hundred thirty and one half pounds.

When Paul lumbered onto the platform a chuckle rippled through the crowd. He was heavy-set, to put it politely, and was barefoot. But the chuckling became stunned silence when he requested over four hundred pounds. Without pretense or hesitation Paul went to the rack and rammed the weight into the air. Footage of this lift shows Paul pressing four hundred two and one half pounds without much visible exertion. Strength records are usually broken by a couple pounds, sometimes fractions of a pound. In an instant Paul bettered the world record by over *seventy* pounds.

Though this was during the Cold War (many felt the American team had been invited just so they could be humiliated), the huge crowd, that included prominent communist party members, leaped to their feat after a moment of shocked silence and roared for several minutes. Paul's feat transcended their politics. Such is the regard Russians have for physical strength.

Showing just how hard Paul trained and how great his ability to gain strength was, two years later he did the same lift with the same weight for <u>seven reps</u>. Later in his career he officially lifted the greatest weight ever lifted overhead with one arm, three hundred eighty pounds, and did three hundred with one arm for ten reps. You can begin to see how he made a two armed single with four hundred two pounds look easy.

The year following the Moscow meet Paul competed in the Olympics in Australia. In spite of being very sick that evening with a one hundred four degree fever, he performed at record level and brought home a gold medal, the last American super heavyweight to do so. My friend Morgan Norval, an old hand in gyms in my area, Marine, author, and holder of several weight lifting records himself, recalls that during these Olympics Paul went down to the track where the U.S. runners were checking out the facilities and 'someone' jokingly suggested a contest in the hundred yard dash between him and one of the world-class sprinters present. To everyone's surprise Paul agreed. When the starting signal came Paul shot off and held the lead for the first fifty yards. The sprinter did overtake him at that point, but consider that Paul then tipped the scales at three hundred thirty pounds, and had been ill with the flu! Morgan doesn't recall the name of the sprinter but perhaps someone reading this does and will provide me the answer.

His official record in the squat was twelve hundred six pounds, and he once did twelve hundred for two reps before witnesses. He often did sets of ten reps with eight hundred pounds, cold with no stretch or warm up. (Do I need to say this? **DON'T**!! Not with <u>any</u> weight) The legendary strongman and bodybuilder John Grimek once witnessed him do a set of ten "quickly" with nine hundred pounds. Paul could do half squats with fourteen hundred pounds, quarter squats with <u>eighteen hundred</u>. He did an absolutely incredible five hundred sixty-five pounds in a very difficult lift no longer done called the jerk press, an all time world record, and bench-pressed six hundred twenty seven pounds. He said he'd benched "a bit more" while not in competition. I've been told that when squatting Paul would sometimes say he was going to do 'a bit more', then add another hundred pounds to the bar. Others have said that Paul was actually a little embarrassed that he wasn't "a strong bencher"(!).

Some of his records have been broken in recent years but there is one that is unlikely to ever be topped. He was in the book of world records for the most weight ever lifted by a human being. It was an exhibition lift, a strength stunt basically, called a back lift, and not a regulation power lift or Olympic lift. Still, this doesn't detract from the fact that he lifted **six thousand two hundred seventy pounds.** To give you a real-life comparison: I drive a full-size sedan. It weighs only three thousand four hundred pounds.

Although he discussed method and technique with his friend Bob Peoples, another champion weightlifter, Paul never had a strength coach or trainer. He believed that strength was the most important factor in weightlifting, when the buzz of the time was that it was "mostly technique" and his training regimen ran contrary to all accepted practice. For example, Paul would train in a single lift or motion with very heavy weight *all day long*. He also knew that leg, hip and back strength were key to overall power at a time when this was thought to have little value. He trained himself on an interesting bunch of home-made equipment, such as a *three thousand pound* safe with a chain and harness he used to do hip bends with, and heavy barbells hanging by chains from great tree limbs that he'd stand beneath to do presses and half presses. One famous photo shows a young Paul ready to squat with a pair of steel tractor wheels dependent from a bar across his shoulders.

I know what some of you are thinking, so let me state right here unequivocally: When Paul started his lifting career anabolic steroids were unknown outside of Soviet veterinary laboratories, and lifting supersuits wouldn't be invented for decades. The only lifting aid he used regularly was a leather lifting belt, although he did once use special hook attachments to pull a one thousand pound deadlift. Of course his official eight hundred twenty pound deadlift was done with bare hands. In competition he was usually barefoot, and he performed most of his exhibition lifts in street clothes, usually jeans and cowboy boots. His anabolic 'secret' was whole milk, and he consumed gallons of it as he trained. He also experimented with various types of protein, notably that derived from peanuts, and extracts of raw beef.

I loved it when he'd take a large nail in one hand and jam the point clear through a two by four. He could also leap flatfooted up onto a three foot high table, and run a hundred yard dash in just over eleven seconds.

Paul became a minister, was a tireless Christian soldier and American patriot, but was most devoted to his work with wayward boys at the youth home he and his wife founded in Georgia. He said that his wife Glenda gave them the love and he provided the discipline. I think attention from Paul Anderson could improve the behavior of even the most incorrigible. I've heard testimonies of some of the young men in their care crediting the Andersons with putting them on the right path. More than one said they'd be either dead or in prison if it hadn't been for Paul and Glenda. A reporter that once interviewed Paul was so moved by the big mans' faith and dedication to his youthful charges that he wrote, "He is the strongest man in the world. He also lifts weights."

What I hope to illustrate by recounting these other facets of Pauls' life is that while the gym is a fine place to be, and weight training a very worthwhile thing to do, we all need balance in our lives and to work at being well-rounded individuals. Paul was stronger than anyone and trained daily, yet much of his time was dedicated to helping others. If you neglect friends, family, and other pursuits and responsibilities of a full and useful life to spend time in the gym, you are training too much. This is another and actually more important definition of overtraining.

Another man of whom mention <u>must</u> be made is Jack LaLanne. Jack was almost single-handedly responsible for the birth of the fitness industry and all of us in it owe him a huge debt. He opened the first modern health club in this country in 1936 and began one of the earliest health club chains as well. He developed some of the first weight training machines, which became prototypes for many of the machines commonly seen in gyms today. The leg extension machine, for example, is an invention of his. Did you ever do a jumping jack? Ever wonder how they got their name? Yep, they are named for Jack LaLanne. He espoused the benefits of natural foods, supplements, and weight training decades before almost anyone else, and anyone who watched television from 1951 to 1985 should remember his pioneering exercise show. Yes, it was on for thirty-four years, a pretty good run by anyones reckoning.

He hit the gym every day at five AM to lift and swim for two hours and claimed to have not missed a workout in *over seventy years*. He dismissed old age as "a myth". To prove this, every year on the occasion of his birthday he performed an incredible feat of strength and endurance. One I recall vividly was on his seventieth birthday when he towed a string of **seventy** small boats, with a reporter in each one, for a mile and a half across Long Beach Harbor while *handcuffed*. He had a standing offer of ten thousand dollars to *anyone* who could keep up with him in one of his workouts. Lou Ferrigno and Arnold Schwarzenegger both tried. It was never earned.

He could do pushups with his weight supported on his toes and fingertips with arms extended straight out past his head. (I challenge you to do <u>one</u> of these – I don't care how old you are). On his ninety-fifth birthday he performed ninety-five pushups on a popular nationally televised talk show. He remained a lifelong picture of strength and radiant health and shortly before he passed away at ninety-six he was still touring the country doing motivational speaking and touting the benefits of a fitness lifestyle. See you again in that big gym upstairs someday Jack.

I know two very strong men (one holds a state bench press record, the other was Mr. Florida for a time), who swear that the strongest man they ever knew was Frank Marcellas. According to them he had twenty-two inch upper arms and was steroid free. Like Paul Anderson he drank great quantities of milk to build size and strength (hard gainers take a note here). He was one of very few people that could press the Louis Cyr dumbbell, weighing two hundred eighty pounds, overhead with one arm. Even more amazingly, Frank could press a three hundred pound barbell straight up overhead, drop it, and *catch it behind his back.* Kids, do not try this at home! Frank also loved to surf and when not working out was usually at the beach. Interestingly, and again just like Paul Anderson, Frank also became a minister.

The Cyr dumbbell, like the Apollon dumbbell, is extremely difficult to press not just because of its weight but because of its huge oversized bar. Even very strong men can't pick it up because they can't get a grip on it. One of the few besides Frank that did was the legendary strength and physique star, John Grimek. In recent years it has been lifted by Mark Henry. Shockingly, it was also lifted by Sig Klein, who weighed only one hundred fifty pounds!

Marvin Eder, barely out of his teens, and at one hundred ninety-eight pounds, did a parallel bar dip bearing an extra *four hundred thirty-four pounds.* Later he was able to do eight parallel bar dips with four hundred pounds fastened to him, and eight wide grip chins with an extra two hundred pounds. Legendary powerlifter Pat Casey, the first man to bench over six hundred pounds and first to squat eight hundred, said that pound for pound Eder was the strongest man to walk the earth.

Two hundred pound Mike Dayton could break police handcuffs, snap baseball bats and police nightsticks, bend pistol barrels, broke a shotgun in half, crushed three cinder blocks at once with a hand strike, and bend coins in half. He chinned himself over eighty times in competition and once popped a basketball. More than once he put a bend in a one inch steel lifting bar. He is a champion bodybuilder and master of more than one form of martial art. Think he can take a blow? He allowed a one hundred twenty three pound girl to jump feetfirst onto his stomach from sixteen feet up, and a two hundred pound man from ten feet up. Imagine sparring with him!

At sixty-seven years old, Curd Edmonds, a student of Mike Dayton's, could chin himself one hundred and twenty times. With wrist straps he could chin himself over two hundred times, and so could his son Chris.

In 1927 Herman Gorner deadlifted seven hundred twenty seven and one half pounds with no straps or hook attachments, to full lockout. Oh yes, he did this with one hand.

Bruce White, an Australian strong man, could chin himself *by grasping two rafters in a pinch grip between thumb and fingers, bearing seventy extra pounds.*

There are so many others that I'd love to write about that this chapter could easily grow larger than the rest of the manual. I will at least mention some more names here, all people whom have performed awesome feats of strength. If this type of history interests you I suggest you look up:

Chuck Ahrens, Vasili Alexiev, Ted Arcidi, 'Professor' Attila, 'Professor' Anthony Barker, Horace Barre, Bourette, Anthony Clark, Ed Coan, Chief Ironbear Collins, Chris Confessore, Slim Farman, Bev Francis, Gary Frank, Arthur Giroux, Joe Greenstein, George Hackenschmidt, Shane Hamman, Jamie Harris, Arthur Hennig, Doug Hepburn, George Jowett, Kirk Karwoski, Bill Kazmaier, Greg Kovacs, John Grunn Marx, Scott Mendelson, Karl Norberg, Arthur Saxon, Becca Swanson, Larry Pacifico, Jan Pall Sigmarsson, Chuck Sipes, Henry 'Milo' Steinborn, Terry Todd, Warren Lincoln Travis, Louis Uni (Apollon), Jack Walsh, Bruce Wilhelm. There are more that are worthy but I can't list them all.

There is a very good chance that the strongest people were or are unknown; perhaps some nameless Canadian lumberjack, anonymous Russian farmer, forgotten Viking giant, or an African quarryman, Scottish highlander, Basque shepherd or old time Mississippi River boatman. All of these backgrounds have produced people of incredible strength.

Maybe, and I hope that this is true, the Paul Anderson of

the twenty-first century is just now picking up weights and thrilling to the feel of moving the heavy iron for the first time. He is probably a burly young lad, an endo-mesomorph, of about thirteen or fourteen years of age, naturally strong by virtue of his body structure, just finding out he loves getting even stronger, and that he's good at it.

But of all the amazing feats of strength, muscle endurance, and power that I know of, one in particular stands out. Many years ago I read a true account of a man who worked in a deep mine when some type of disaster struck. He and several other men were trapped on an elevator platform that stalled in the shaft as a result. They were in immediate danger from gas, fire, or maybe collapse of the mine. At any rate, this man *climbed up the elevator cables with a coworker on his back nearly a hundred feet to safety, then went back down the cable and repeated this until he had rescued all the men on the elevator.*

If you don't comprehend what a mind-boggling feat this is, I'll put it in perspective for you. Remember the climbing rope in gym class? There was always some athletic kid who could do it and make it look easy, but generally making it to the top of the rope and down again was *tough*, impossible even, for many of us, and it was no more than fifteen to twenty feet high.

Now imagine making this climb on a dirty, greasy, perhaps frayed, steel cable about five times that length, at least six times up and five times down. On the trips down you must of course support your own bodyweight, but on the trips up the cable you must climb supporting not only your own but also that of another man on your back. If you fail, you, the man you're carrying, and all those still below will die. If you even stop to rest, all those men will die. Ponder that one for awhile. I say with no shame that it makes me feel small.

I've searched my archives but am unable to come up with the name of this hero as of this writing, but this is the most miraculous feat of strength and muscle endurance that I've ever heard of. With due respect to all the strong men and women I have mentioned, the lifting of inanimate hunks of iron, no matter how massive, pales in comparison to this.

YOUR RESPONSIBILITY

When I'd developed some significant strength and put on some size, Bear Dickerson, with a surprising concern and gentleness that big men sometimes show, sat me down to tell me in no uncertain terms that strength comes with a price tag.

I thought he meant all the hours of sweat and torturous effort in the gym, and all the days of sore, stiff muscles, and I wondered out loud why he felt I needed to be reminded of this.

"Thats not what I mean." He ran a huge meaty hand through his hair and sighed. "There's a big responsibility that comes along with strength. A responsibility to **not** use it." He didn't mean in the gym.

The lightbulb finally came on. "Oh. You mean against someone else."

"That's it."

I understood then precisely where he was coming from. He and I had been in the Marine Corps together, we were bikers in those days, patronized some seedy dives now and again, and had what many considered a rough and rowdy lifestyle. He's also one of very few people who have seen me get really angry. Aside from being a mighty strong three hundred fifteen pound man, Bear had grown up in an exceptionally rough part of Philadelphia during an exceptionally rough time, and had also been a martial arts instructor. I deferred to him in matters like these. Still do.

He went on to relate an account of a powerlifter he'd trained with, forced to defend himself against two other big men in a barroom brawl, who used his great strength and street fighting experience to end the altercation in a very decisive manner. He was charged with attempted murder due to the extensive and serious injuries he inflicted on his foes, <u>even though</u> the court acknowledged that he had been attacked, was outnumbered, and was defending himself. The prosecutor said he had used 'excessive force', and put forth the argument that he was also guilty of assault with a deadly weapon, i.e. his massive and enormously strong body.

"They were talking about a long time behind bars for my friend. Cost him a lot of time and money to get out of that fix but he finally did, thank God." Bears next words still ring in my ears from time to time. "I'd hate to see you in a predicament like that because you don't know your own strength, or aren't mature enough to keep from using it in the wrong way."

Good strong words from a good strong man.

See you in the gym!